Translation Studies and Eye-Tracking Analysis

Warschauer Studien zur Germanistik und zur Angewandten Linguistik

Herausgegeben von Sambor Grucza und Lech Kolago

Band 6

PETER LANG EDITION

Sambor Grucza / Monika Płużyczka /
Justyna Zając (eds)

Translation Studies and Eye-Tracking Analysis

PETER LANG
EDITION

Bibliographic Information published by the Deutsche Nationalbibliothek
The Deutsche Nationalbibliothek lists this publication in the Deutsche Nationalbibliografie; detailed bibliographic data is available in the internet at http://dnb.d-nb.de.

The publication was financially supported by University of Warsaw Faculty of Applied Linguistics Institute of Anthropocentric Linguistics and Culturology University of Warsaw Foundation

FUNDACJA UNIWERSYTETU WARSZAWSKIEGO

All the books published in the series are reviewed before publication.

Editorial support: Jadwiga Marczyk, M.A., Marta Najman, M.A.

Cover Design: © Olaf Gloeckler, Atelier Platen, Friedberg

Library of Congress Cataloging-in-Publication Data

Translation studies and eye-tracking analysis / Sambor Grucza, Monika Płużyczka, Justyna Zając (eds).
pages cm. — (Warschauer Studien Zur Germanistik Und Zur Angewandten Linguistik ; Band 6)
Includes bibliographical references.
ISBN 978-3-631-63448-6
1. Translating and interpreting—Research. 2. Eye—Movements—Research. 3. Visual communication—Technique. 4. Visual communication—Research. I. Grucza, Sambor, editor of compilation.
P306.2.T7345 2013
418'.02072—dc23

2013010035

ISSN 2192-7820
ISBN 978-3-631-63448-6

Peter Lang Edition is an Imprint of Peter Lang GmbH.

Peter Lang – Frankfurt am Main · Bern · Bruxelles · New York · Oxford · Warszawa · Wien

www.peterlang.de

Table of Contents

Eye-Tracking Supported Translation Studies at the University of Warsaw (Instead of Introduction)

Sambor Grucza, Monika Płużyczka, Justyna Zając
(University of Warsaw)

The results of thoughts and discussions, and eye-tracking supported research carried out within the scope of broadly understood translation studies at the Faculty of Applied Linguistics at the University of Warsaw by a team from the Linguistics of Languages for Specific Purposes Department gave rise to this volume.

Scientific research concerning specialized languages, and textual and discursive representation of specialized knowledge constitute the primary objective of the Department. These research objectives are realized in two areas – descriptive/explicative and applicative, and concern English, German, Polish and Russian specialized languages. Descriptive/explicative tasks aim to determine the expression exponents of specific thinking and/or of speaking about what a given (investigated) representative of a given specialist community or a researched subset of its representatives does, in other words, to determine the specific language of his/her work, the object of this work and its results (see A. Bajerowska 2011; S. Grucza 2012a, 2012b, 2012e). Applicative tasks concern both, reflections on the future (development) of specialized languages, as well as thoughts on the development of (linguistic) research into specialized languages. The former attempt to first answer the question of how the researched specialized languages naturally develop, i.e. development which takes place with no external interference, and then whether there is a possibility to rationally interfere in the development of specialized languages in order to improve the specialized languages researched in this way, and to master the skill of using them, and finally the question of how one can enhance specialized discourses, i.e. the use of specialized texts, namely, to enhance specialized languages in such a way that it would enable specialists using them to fulfil their needs and/or objectives, both cognitive and communicative, the best they can (for more on that see S. Grucza 2012a). Our research includes, amongst other things, applicative research into pilot–air traffic control tower communication, carried out by Anna P. Borowska, PhD (2011, 2012) and research into business communication, carried out by Justyna Zając, PhD (2012a, 2012b, 2012c, 2012d).

The Department also researches languages/specialized texts within the field of glottodidactics and translation studies. The primary glotodidactic tasks of the Department are conducted under the aegis of the LISTiG scientific project, which aims to produce effective, linguistically-intelligent software that contains standard didactic modules covering the field of Polish-German language problems, connected to selected specialized languages (see S. Grucza 2010a, 2010b, 2010c, 2010d, 2012c, 2012e; S. Grucza et al. 2012; P. Szerszeń 2010, 2011, 2012; and A. Dickiel 2010, 2011).

Within the field of translation studies, experimentally-oriented research is carried out into pure translation studies investigating translation processes, as well as into applied linguistics, mainly into translodidactics. Experimental eye-tracking supported research into translation processes was initiated at the Linguistics of Languages for Specific Purposes Department as early as the beginning of 2011. The first eye-tracking experiments were carried out thanks to 'eyetracking.pl', which was so kind as to make a Tobii T120 eye-tracker available to members of the Department. The first observations and remarks relating to the experiments were published in 2011 (see S. Grucza 2012d, 2012e; M. Płużyczka 2011a, 2011b, 2012a, 2012b; E. Plewa 2011; E. Zwierzchoń-Grabowska 2011).

In 2012, the Ministry of Science and Higher Education allocated a scientific grant to Professor Sambor Grucza and Monika Płużyczka, PhD for the purpose of purchasing equipment. This enabled the purchase of an SMI RED 500 eye-tracker and the establishment of the Eye-Tracking Experimental Linguistics Laboratory (LELO). This is the first eye-tracking laboratory in the history of Polish Linguistics, which aims to carry out systematic glottodidactic and translation studies-oriented experimental research. The laboratory research team under scientific supervision by professor Sambor Grucza includes Monika Płużyczka, PhD (research supervision), Justyna Zając, PhD, Ewa Zwierzchoń-Grabowska, PhD, Anna Kudłaj M.A. and Marta Najman, M.A. It should be added that eye-tracking research at the Faculty of Linguistics is also carried out by A. Szarkowska, Ph.D., whose main research interest is audio-visual translation, in particular audio-description.

The primary task of LELO is to carry out research within experimental eye-tracking supported linguistics, in particular within eye-tracking supported translation studies and glottodidactics, verifying and complementing their previous findings. Currently, two areas of interest within specialized text translation studies are being subjected to experimental eye-tracking supported research: (1) the process of sight translation of specialized texts, and (2) the process of audio-visual translation. Within the field of glottodidactics regarding specialized texts, experimental eye-tracking supported research should focus on:

(1) the process of specialized text reading, and (2) the process of reconstructing/creating specialized knowledge. All the tasks undertaken concern both descriptive translation studies and translodidactics equally.

This publication presents the results of our research and scientific experiments. However, this is not our only goal, since this publication aims, on the one hand to outline the theoretical foundations on which our experimental research is based, while on the other hand, to present a slightly broader range of questions to be asked/answered by eye-tracking supported translation studies. Therefore, the texts have been arranged into two thematic, though not formally distinct parts. The first part includes texts dedicated to the theoretical foundations of translation studies-oriented eye-tracking research, while the other includes texts discussing the results of the experiments that were carried out.

The first part opens the paper by **Sambor Grucza**, *Heat Maps, Gaze Plots ... and What Next? The Access to Translation Competences and Translation Process*. It comprises two main parts. The first part of the paper concentrates on the translation competences and it draws a distinction between idiocompetences and polycompetences. This division is followed by differentiation between two types of translation studies, which allows to focus on the studies of real translation competences and the objectives of real translation studies. The second part elaborates on the term 'text' in relation to the translation competences, translation studies and the possibility to reconstruct translation competence by means of text analysis. Since the translation competence is embedded in human brain, these deliberations are followed by presenting the aspects of cognition and the concept of equipment-based cognition and its limitations, culminating in the eye-tracking method as the most effective research method of translation process.

Jerzy Żmudzki's paper *Problems, Objectives and Challenges of the Polish Translation Studies and Theory* undertakes all the issues addressed in its title, brings up the remarks, fears and difficulties of the academic translators' society. The article begins with the description of distinguishable phases of the translation theory development in Poland, followed by references to the illustrious publications. The paper lists Polish universities conducting extensive research in the field of translation and interpreting, and mentions the types of problems that are yet to be overcome by the scholars, for instance institutionalisation and institutional diversity, involvement in various conferences and organisations, terminological diversity in separate departments and unilateral understanding of the theory of translation. The article also covers the challenges concerning translation didactics. The paper finishes with the description of the issues affecting the state exam for sworn translators.

The paper *Knowledge – Transference – Translation* by **Marta Małachowicz** focuses on presenting three title concepts and relations existing between them. The article underlines the importance of the correct understanding of these terms and cautions the reader against confusing their academic meaning with the literal sense. The definitions of knowledge, transference and translation are discussed within the anthropocentric approach to language and communication, which means putting human beings in the central position and concentrating on the abilities and potentials of their brains. The most emphasized issues are the transference and transference acts that are the starting point of the knowledge popularization process and are immensely important for communication. Transference of knowledge that is specific for a new domain is usually accompanied by transference of new expressional means from source language to target language, which is of great importance especially for the translators of specialist texts.

The article *Eye-Tracking Methods and Measures* by **Paweł Soluch** and **Adam Tarnowski** complexly covers the topic of eyeball movements which can be described as the commonest potentially intentional human behaviour. The observations during reading have been carried out by scholars for centuries, yet nowadays due to the technological development it is possible to introduce far more accurate and advanced eye-tracking devices. The paper describes thoroughly the perception process, differentiates types of eye movements, then moves on to the mechanisms that ensure the stability of perception and comments on modern methods of measurement of eyeball movement. The article underlines that eye-trackers have already been applied to various areas of life and science, like linguistics, psychology or law, just to name a few. The current studies in the field of eye-tracking concentrate mostly on the cognitive processes behind the eye movement. Eye-tracking research has been experiencing a growing interest, yet the topic demands even more attention and exploration as a vast and fertile branch of knowledge.

The aim of the article of **Ewa Zwierzchoń-Grabowska**, *Could Eye-Tracking Help to Reconstruct the Translation Processes?*, is to present the possibilities of application of eye-tracking methodology to the research of interlanguage translation. The development of non-invasive methods for measuring eye motion and computer technologies allows researchers to record and analyze a huge volume of data that eye movement generates. Thus, eye-tracking research expands intensively. The first part of the article presents selected types of interlanguage translation and the possibilities of their testing with a video eye-tracker. The second part of the article focuses on participants in video eye-tracking research.

The second part of the book begins with the article by **Monika Płużyczka** *Eye-Tracking Supported Research Into Sight Translation. Lapsological Conclusions*. It presents the significance of eye-tracking experimental research in translation studies and translation didactics. The main parts of the article describe and comment on an experiment conducted among a group of a professional interpreter and sixteen students, who were to sight translate a short text from Polish (mother tongue) into Russian (first or second foreign language). The study aimed to analyse the cognitive possibilities of eye-tracking research in translation studies, to observe the process of translation and to formulate conclusions concerning the translodidactic relevance of eye-tracking research. The results of the experiment are described thoroughly and are coupled with corresponding heatmaps and gaze plots. The article ends with the conclusions regarding usefulness of eye-tracking research for translation didactics.

The article *Proactive Use of Eye Tracking in the Translational Workflow* by **Silvia Hansen-Schirra** and **Christoph Rösener** describes new ideas and proposals related to the use of gaze-assisted interaction in modern translation. The paper discusses software applications used in the translational workflow, taking into consideration the distinction between three stages of the translation process – before, during and after translation – and possible modifications that aim to improve this interactions. In the following part an interpretation of some-eye tracking data recorded during translation process is presented, as well as scenarios of applying different terminology workflow, namely: bilingual word clouds, translation memory systems (SDL Trados Studio and OmegaT) and corpus data. Each method is analyzed from the efficiency perspective and ability to make text processing more productive. The studies discussed in the article may help in further improvements of the translation practice and the translational workflow.

Agnieszka Szarkowska, Izabela Krejtz, Krzysztof Krejtz and **Andrew Duchowski** present in their paper *Harnessing the Potential of Eye-Tracking for Media Accessibility* an overview of eye-tracking research studies in the area of media accessibility. The paper begins with a description of eye-tracking methodology and studies that use eye movement behaviour to investigate cognitive processes. The main part of the article presents four studies carried out by its authors: the first one concentrates on providing subtitles for the deaf and hard of hearing, and is a part of the DTV4ALL project; the second study deals with subtitles on digital television for the same group of recipients; the third and the fourth studies undertake the issue of audio description for the blind and partially sighted in education and in art respectively. The results of the research can be implemented in the audiovisual translation professional market practices and in education.

The second experimental part discussing the results of the experiments that were carried out ends with the article *Eye-Tracking Research of Business Email Reception* by **Justyna Zając**. The author compares selected results from the qualitative study of business email discourse conducted within a particular global project team, with eye-tracking data from emailers' actual reactions. The findings discussed concern the initiating of business email discourse and business email titles. The first part of her paper presents some aspects of current business practice (project management, geocentric approach to staffing) and the main linguistics characteristics of business (email) discourse in international settings. The second part describes the study (data, methods, data donor), and focuses on discussing the results of the receipt of business email that initiates specialist discourse, and business email titles. The article finishes with suggestions for possible future studies on business email discourse.

References

Bajerowska, A. (2011): *Antropocentryczna a korelatywne koncepcje wiedzy i informacji.* In: Lingwistyka Stosowana/ Applied Linguistics/ Angewandte Linguistik. 4. 229–239.

Borowska, A. P. (2011): *O konieczności usprawnienia procesu akwizycji lotniczego języka angielskiego na tle antropocentrycznej teorii języka.* In: Cz. Dyrcz (ed.), Bezpieczeństwo w portach lotniczych i morskich. Zeszyty Naukowe AMW Nr 186A. Gdynia. 7–12.

Borowska, A. P. (2012): *Usprawnienie komunikacji pilot–wieża: zadanie dla lingwistyki języków specjalistycznych.* In: Lingwistyka Stosowana/ Applied Linguistics/ Angewandte Linguistik. 5. 19–29.

Dickel, A. (2010): *Bestimmung des Sprachmaterials für den Fachsprachenunterricht Wirtschaftsdeutsch für angehende Dolmetscher/ Übersetzer.* In: A. Małgorzewicz (ed.), Translation: Teorie – Praxis – Didaktik. Wrocław. 293–301.

Dickel, A. (2011): *Didaktik des Fachsprachenunterrichts.* In: Komunikacja Specjalistyczna. 5. 1–25.

Grucza, S. (2010a): *Sprache(n) – Fachsprache(n) – Fachsprachendidaktik.* In: G. Łopuszańska (ed.), Studien zur sprachlichen Kommunikation. Gdańsk. 31–46.

Grucza, S. (2010b): *Specyfika uczenia języków specjalistycznych w świetle antropocentrycznej teorii języka.* In: A. Waszczuk-Zin (ed.), Lingwistyka stosowana – języki specjalistyczne – dyskurs zawodowy. Warszawa. 107–130.

Grucza, S. (2010c): *Glottodydaktyka specjalistyczna – jej przedmiot i cele poznawcze.* In: J. Knieja/ T. Zygmunt/ Ł. Brzana (eds), Literaturoznawstwo, językoznawstwo i kulturoznawstwo jako płaszczyzny przekazu we współczesnej glottodydaktyce. Lublin. 35–48.

Grucza, S. (2010d): *Język a poznanie – kilka uwag na temat rozważania ich wzajemnych relacji.* In: S. Grucza/ A. Marchwiński/ M. Płużyczka (eds), Translatoryka. Koncepcje – Modele – Analizy. Warszawa. 54–67.

Grucza, S. (2012a): *Fachsprachenlinguistik.* Frankfurt/ M.

Grucza, S. (2012b): *Ścisłość języków specjalistycznych a ścisłość tekstów specjalistycznych*. In: K. Grzywka/ R. Małecki/ M. Filipowicz/ J. Godlewicz-Adamiec/ P. Kociumbas/ D. Wyrzykiewicz/ E. Michta (ed.), Kultura – literatura – język. Pogranicza Komparatystyki./ Kultur – Literatur – Sprache. Warszawa. 1272–1285.

Grucza, S. (2012c): *Zum Begriff „didaktischer Text" in der Fachtranslationsdidaktik*. In: M. Olpińska–Szkiełko/ S. Grucza/ Z. Berdychowska/ J. Żmudzki (eds), Der Mensch und seine Sprachen. Frankfurt/ M. 254–271.

Grucza, S. (2012d): *The Investigation of Translation Competences and Translation Processes*. In: Vestnik MGLU (in press).

Grucza, S. (2012e): *Kognitive Funktion von Fachsprachen als Gegenstand der Fachsprachenlinguistik*. In: F. Grucza/ H.-R. Spiegel/ O. Schneider-Mizony/ J. Żmudzki (eds), Akten des XII. internationalen Germanistenkongresses, Warschau 2010. Fachsprachen in Theorie und Praxis. Geschichte des Deutschen als Fremdsprachenunterricht weltweit/ Geschichte von DaF weltweit. Theorie und Geschichte der Translationswissenschaft. Bd. 18. Frankfurt/ M. 31–37.

Grucza, S./ A. Dickel/ U. Burda/ P. Szerszeń (2012), *LISTiG – Wsparcie e-learningowe dla praktyki glotto- i translodydaktycznej*, (w:) Lingwistyka Stosowana/ Applied Linguistics/ Angewandte Linguistik 6, 59-74

Hryniuk, K. (2011): *Okulograficzne wsparcie badań nad procesem czytania*. In: Lingwistyka Stosowana/ Applied Linguistics/ Angewandte Linguistik. 4. 191–198.

Plewa, E. (2011): *Okulograficzne wsparcie badań nad procesem tłumaczenia audiowizualnego*. In: Lingwistyka Stosowana/ Applied Linguistics/ Angewandte Linguistik. 4. 211–220.

Płużyczka, M. (2010): *Wybrane trudności translacyjne a proces translodydaktyczny*. In: S. Piotrowski (ed.), O nauczaniu i uczeniu się języka obcego dla potrzeb zawodowych. Lublin. 88–97.

Płużyczka, M. (2011a): *Okulograficzne wsparcie badań nad procesem tłumaczenia a vista*. In: Lingwistyka Stosowana/ Applied Linguistics/ Angewandte Linguistik. 4. 181–189.

Płużyczka, M. (2011b): *Eye-Tracking Analysen in der Translatorik. Zum Stand der Forschung*. In: Kwartalnik Neofilologiczny. LVIII. 4/ 2011. 11–23.

Płużyczka, M. (2012a): *Eye-Tracking Support of Translation Processes Analysis*. In: Vestnik MGLU, Moskwa (in press).

Płużyczka, M. (2012b): *Na co patrzy, a co widzi tłumacz a vista? Okulograficzne pytania translatoryki*. In: Lingwistyka Stosowana/ Applied Linguistics/ Angewandte Linguistik. 5. 65–74.

Szerszeń, P. (2010): *Glottodydaktyka a (hiper)teksty internetowe*. Warszawa.

Szerszeń, P. (2011): *Glottodidaktische Bewertung der deutschsprachigen Internetfachtexte für den DaF–Fachsprachenunterricht an polnischen (Hoch)Schulen am Beispiel einer Textanalyse aus dem Bereich Wirtschaft*. In: Orbis Linguarum. 25–30.

Szerszeń, P. (2012): *Zum Stand der Fachsprachendidaktikforschung in Polen. Ein Abriss*. In: M. Olpińska-Szkiełko/ S. Grucza/ Z. Berdychowska/ J. Żmudzki (eds), Der Mensch und seine Sprachen. Frankfurt/ M. 587–596.

Zwierzchoń-Grabowska, E. (2011): *Okulograficzne wsparcie badań nad tłumaczeniem pisemnym*. In: Lingwistyka Stosowana/ Applied Linguistics/ Angewandte Linguistik. 4. 199–210.

Zając, J. (2012a): *Specialist Email Communication in Global Virtual Teams: Selected Facets of Politeness*. (11th Annual Conference of the European Association of Languages for Specific Purposes: „The Role of Applied Languages in Tertiary Education in the post – Bologna scenario: boosting autonomy and mobility in a globalised world?". (in press)

Zając, J. (2012b): *Linguistic Issues of Email Discourse in Business Communication*. In: Studia Germanica Gedanensia. 26. 235–246.

Zając, J. (2012c): *Towards Successful Communication in Global Virtual Teams: Team Language and Team Culture*. In: Kwartalnik Neofilologiczny. LIX. 3/ 2012. 345–370.

Zając, J. (2012d): *Communication in Global Corporations. Successful Project Management via Email*. Frankfurt/ M. (forthcoming).

Heat Maps, Gaze Plots . . . and What Next? The Access to Translation Competences and Translation Processes

Sambor Grucza (University of Warsaw)

Introduction

For some time already, a discourse within the field of translation studies has increasingly focused on the translator, his/her translation properties and mental processes resulting from their application. Recent years and advances in technology, have opened up many possibilities of gaining a deeper insight into these processes (see S. Grucza 2011). In the first part of this article I shall characterize the object of translation studies and attempt to introduce the possibilities of its cognition (cf. S. Grucza 2010). In the second part, I shall briefly present the capabilities and limitations of equipment-based cognition in translation studies, with particular emphasis on the applicability of eye-tracking research to translation studies.

1. Translation competences

Real translation competences are located in the human brain. What it means is that no translation competence, nor any other type of competence for that matter, is available for direct observation. Competence models, on the other hand, are intellectual generalizations, idealizations, models of a particular set of real competences. Therefore, to begin with, a distinction should be made between real translation competences and translation competence models and then, between the reconstructions (descriptions) of actual translation competences and idealized translation competences models.

This implies that the designata of the term 'translation competence' should be categorized into the following two groups (a) real translation competences i.e. the competences of particular translators (idiocompetences) and (b) intellectual constructs, the ideal models of the first group (polycompetences). The polylectal area can be illustrated in the following way:

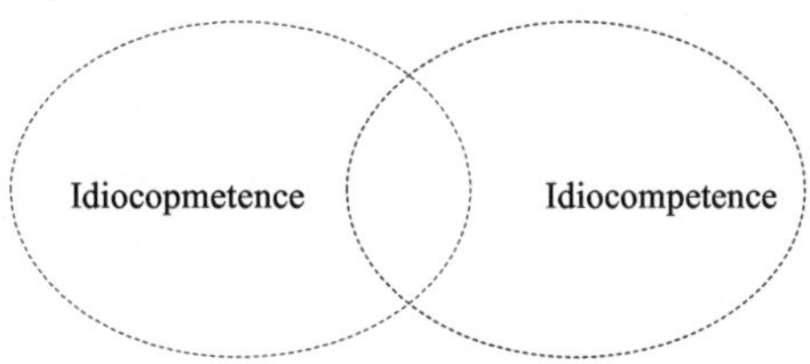

Fig. 1: *Polycompetence: intersection or logical sum*

Consequently, a primary division of translation competences calls for, as previously stated, a division of translation studies into translation studies investigating real translation competences – translation studies concerning real languages, and translation studies investigating these generalizations, (intellectual) constructs (models), ideal models (descriptions) of translation competences – competence model linguistics. Undoubtedly, the primacy of real competences translation studies should be recognized, as their results provide a necessary basis for rational deliberation on competence models translation studies.

Making a distinction between the two types of translation studies (translation studies investigating real translation competences and translation studies researching models of translation competences – generating and/or perfecting them) is, in view of our debate, essential, since issues relating to their material, objects and objectives differ. Subsequently, I will shift to some issues pertaining to studies of real translation competences, which, henceforth, I shall refer to as 'anthropocentric translation studies', in short, 'translation studies'.

Let us reiterate it: (real) translation competences are located in the brains of (particular) translators. This means that any competence (idiocompetance) cognition can only be arrived at through the observation and analysis of behaviours as well as products (the results) of particular translation operations performed by a competence possessor, that is to say a particular translator, in particular through the analysis of (a) his/her received and produced (being produced) utterances, and (b) the way s/he uses the former and the latter. These reflections can be illustrated by means of a translation model where TP = Text Producer, T1 = Original, TC = Translation Competence, TP = Translation Process, T2 = Translat, and T2 = Text Recipient.

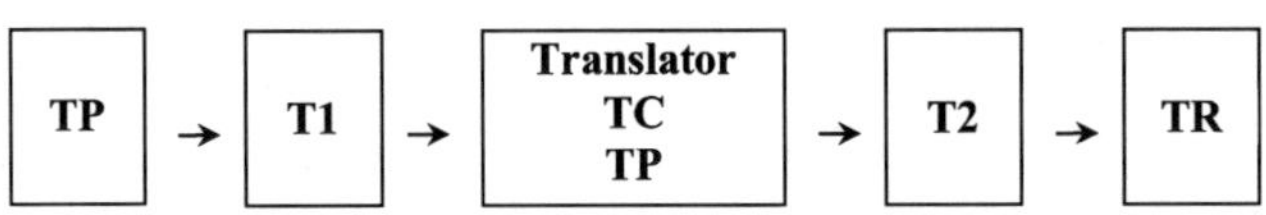

Fig. 2: The holistic Translation Model (S. Grucza 2008, 2012b)

An assumption that the reconstruction of translation competences and the processes resulting from their application is the main purpose of translation studies, gives rise to two fundamental questions: (1) Which of the translator's skills and within what scope should (can) be recognized as translation skills and, (2) Which mental processes and to what extent should (can) be recognized as translation processes? The answers to both these questions have already been formulated previously, however, and for obvious reasons, to a limited degree

(F. Grucza 1981, 1986; B. Z. Kielar 1986, 1988; A. Marchwiński 1993; M. Płużyczka 2008; see also D. Płońska/B. Bokus 2010).

The real translation competences, i.e. the competences of particular translators, can be approached from either a broader or narrower perspective, i.e. the set of competences referred to as translation idiocompetences can be made up of various competences. For the purpose of this debate, I shall assume that the following should be included in translation competences[1]: (a) (bilingual) language ability in a first (native) language (L1) and a second (foreign) language (L2), (b) the ability to carry out a semantic analysis of the text, (c) the ability to discern vital information in T1, (d) the ability to switch from L1 to L2 with a view of expressing the same content in T2, as expressed by the primary text producer in T1, (e) the ability to give T2 a form corresponding to the form of T1, generated by the primary text producer, (f) the ability to professionally transcode the information from L1 to L2 and adjust it to L2 cultural context. Furthermore: (g) the ability to recognize the translation chain, (h) the ability to select an appropriate translation strategy (the ability to carry out appropriate translation processes).

Here, it should also be added that translation idiocompetences of a particular speaker/listener, i.e. of a particular translator, can be approached in two ways: from either an analytic or an ontological point of view. From the analytic point of view translation idiocompetences should be examined as certain isolated self-contained wholes, that is to say, as if they constituted a certain isolated set of particular competences, as if the components of this set were autonomous in relation to other idiocompetences.

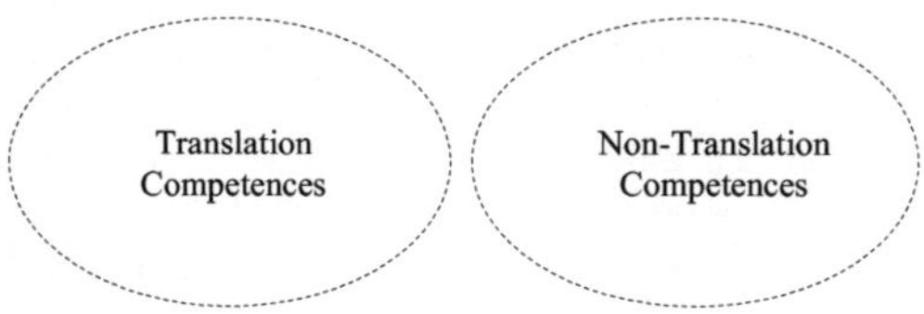

Fig. 3: The analytic approach to translation competences

However, from the ontological point of view, competences included within the set of translation idiocompetences are not autonomous in relation to the other types of idiocompetences of a particular speaker/listener. In other words, the set of translation idiocompetences does not constitute an autonomous set of competences.

1 See F. Grucza 1981, 1986, 1993; B. Z. Kielar 1986, 1988, 2003; A. Marchwiński 1993.

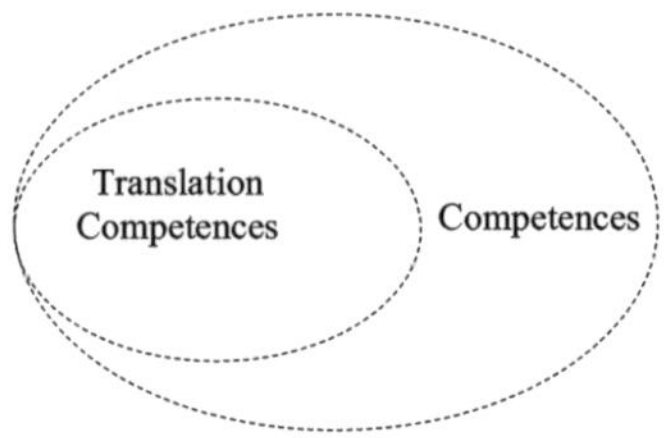

Fig. 4: The ontological approach to translation competences

Competences constituting the set of translation idiocompetences are referred to as language competences, competences to some extent referred to as cultural competences as well as a number of other competences, which, when applied, enable a translator to receive and understand a source text, and subsequently, to convey particular information either in a target text or, alternatively, process this information for the needs of a target recipient and express it appropriately. It is precisely finding the answer to the question of which translator's competences should be included into the set of his/her translation idiocompetences that constitutes one of the main objectives of diagnostic translation studies (for more on this topic see S. Grucza 2012c).

Although exploring the above fundamental questions, (1) which of the translator's skills and within what scope should (can) be recognized as translation skills and, (2) which mental processes and to what extent should (can) be recognized as translation processes, is of utmost difficulty, it should be remembered that:

> What we need to do first is to learn about its subject, i.e., we must first describe that subject, explain its observable properties etc. To set about formulating an answer to the question of how to improve the translation process, which translation methods to apply etc. without first learning about what translation consists of, what operations are performed by a translator, in what sequence, why they are done in this way and in this very sequence and so on, would be like setting the cart before the horse. [...] In fact the main objective of translation theory conceived as a field of inquiry (hence not only as a body of knowledge) is to come to know its subject, i.e., first to describe how matters stand within it, and then to explain why this is the case etc. (F. Grucza 1985: 269).

However, the cognitive objectives of translation studies are not limited solely to the reconstruction (description) of the competences which make up its field of interest. These objectives also include the reconstruction (description) and explication (explanation) of translation processes/operations that take place in the mind of the translator during the act of translation. Incidentally, bearing in mind the issues already put forward, these are the very objectives, i.e. the reconstruction and explication of translation processes, that have been coming up to the fore in translation studies research lately – they are of particular interest to experimentally-oriented translation studies (see *inter alia* S. Grucza 2011, 2012a; M. Płużyczka 2011a, 2011b, 2012a, 2012b). Furthermore, translation studies also aim to research the possibility of finding solutions to the problems that translators are confronted with as well as to research the possibility of optimizing translators' work (for more on that see F. Grucza 1981).

Summing up, let us add to our reflections that in general the objectives of translation studies, as is the case with any scientific discipline for that matter, fall into three categories: diagnostic, anagnostic and prognostic. The objectives with which any empirical science, and therefore translation studies as well, should commence researching its object of cognition are diagnostic objectives; it is a diagnosis. I shall refer to this type of translation studies as pure translation studies, with its objective being to produce a body of knowledge on the translation competences of real translators and translation processes going on in their minds – competences and processes assumed to be observable here and now. Other objectives that translation studies should address are anagnostic objectives (referring to the situation assumed to have existed in the past) and prognostic objectives (referring to the situation assumed/expected to come into existence/to be existing in the future). I shall refer to the former as historical translation studies and to the latter, pertaining to prognostic objectives, as applied translation studies (for more on that topic see S. Grucza 2012c).

To conclude, the relations between the diagnostic, anagnostic and prognostic objectives and the relations between the respective types of translation studies realizing these objectives are presented graphically in Figure 5. The fundamental elements of the in the following Figure defined objectives are the diagnostic objectives, as the body of knowledge produced in the process of their realization constitutes the derivative basis for both anagnostic and prognostic knowledge. However, the anagnostic knowledge, to some extent, complements the diagnostic knowledge as it provides explication of diagnostic findings. Prognostic knowledge, on the other hand, can be looked upon either as a specific continuation of the progressive (running along the time vector) anagnostic perspective or, as a specific antecedent of a regressive anagnostic perspective. Figure 5 illustrates these relations with the use of arrows (for more on that topic see F. Grucza 1981, 1983, 1990):

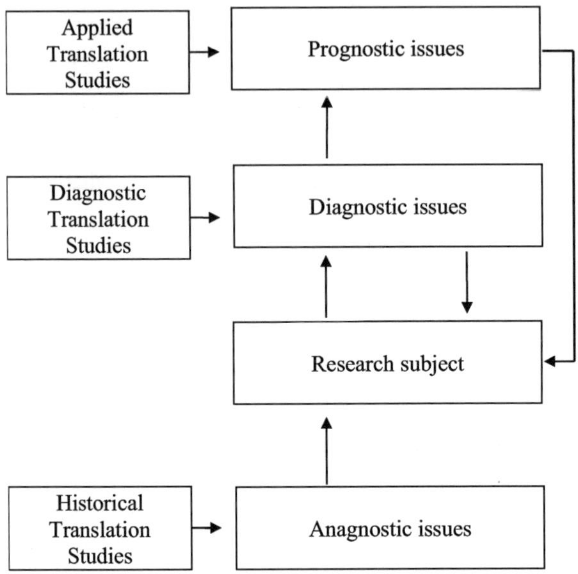

Fig. 5: Issues of Translation Studies

2. Reconstructing translation competence

Let us return to the issue under study. Since any translation competence is not amenable to direct empirical observation, to describe such a translation competence means to 'reconstruct' it, that is to reconstruct a particular translator's relevant (analytical-generative) properties, and especially, to reconstruct the knowledge founding them. Reconstructing the relevant properties of real translators entails determining the 'catalogue' of the factors of their knowledge and/or skills, on the basis of which they have received and understood (or are able to receive and understand) texts in L1 and have produced (or are able to produce) texts in L2, and the factors on the basis of which they are able to express in L2 texts knowledge/information/intentions, as expressed in L1 texts.

G. Toury (1982: 25) when elaborating on the possibilities of translation process cognition referred to the human brain as a 'black box' and wrote:

> Translated texts and their constitutive elements are observational texts […]. Translation processes, those series of operations whereby actual translations are derived from actual source texts, though no doubt also empirical facts, and as such

part of the object-level of translation studies, are nevertheless only indirectly available for study as a kind of 'black box'.

D. Sandra (1998) entering into a discussion with W. Croft on the possibilities of mental representations cognition says: 'Those who propose models of mental representation (or suggest such representation) often commit a fallacy. [...] When discussing mental representations, linguists are more likely to confess a belief than to prove a point' (*ibid.* p. 361). She continues:

> What can linguists learn about human mind by studying language? Let me begin by reiterating what they cannot learn. Linguists cannot address issues pertaining to processing of linguistic material. Such issues concern the language processor rather than the language itself and hence fall outside the limits of linguistic research and within the boundaries of psycholinguistics, which makes use of chronometric techniques for studying ongoing processing. Linguists cannot make statements about the representational format of language elements in the language user's mind either.

And further she adds:

> In contrast, linguists are able to make some statements on what is in the mind. This especially applies to humans' mental predisposition for language, which may be identified through a careful study of what makes languages typically human [...] (*ibid.* p. 375)[2].

Of course, the reconstruction of the translators' appropriate translation properties (competences), does not constitute an easy task. A. R. Luria was right, when writing in 1974 in the first issue of *Language and Brain*:

> The question of the relation of language and brain belongs to the most complex problems in science. The history of attempts to solve it has been replete with confrontations of opposite approaches, often leading to dead ends. A solution to this problem requires a radical revision of our basic concepts, which have remained unchanged for many decades (A. R. Luria 1974: 1).

And thirty five years later G. Benedetti et al. (2009: 1) are made to admit that:

> Despite allowing for the unprecedented visualization of brain functional activity, modern neurobiological techniques have not yet been able to provide satisfactory answers to important questions about the relationship between brain and mind.

It is my duty as a scholar to add that defining factors enabling a translator to perform broadly understood translation activities, constitutes the main objective of translation studies investigating real translators.

As I have already stated, it is translation studies of real translation competences that are of interest to me. As far it is concerned, the statement that particular texts constitute real means of communication implies that, by its

---

2 See also W. G. Raymond/T. Matlock 2000.

nature, translation studies must commence its discussion and research with an analysis of particular texts that are being produced (have been produced) and/or texts that are being received (have been received) in particular acts (processes) of communication. This leads to the conclusion that the particular texts should be recognized as objects, constituting the primary translation studies material. However, the particular texts, on no account, constitute the right object for research studies. This is so because no creators' languages, no translation processes, and what is more, no translation competences are included in the texts. Translation operations are to translation competences as actions are to the skills required to execute them (the actions). And texts are to translation competences as artifacts are to the tools used to produce them. Texts, on the other hand, are to translation operations as artifacts are to the actions undertaken to produce them. This means that one way or another, texts should be recognized as the primary research material for translation studies. And since no texts comprise either a translation competence or translation operation, and what is more, they are not autonomous beings, then, out of necessity, they should be reflected upon and examined in connection with their producers and recipients.

The fact that the reconstruction of translation competences is possible only by means of the analysis of externalized products, i.e. by means of text analysis, makes defining what texts are and what they are not fundamental to translation studies deliberations. This objective should commence with clarifying issues referring, on the one hand, to the expression 'text' and, on the other, to objects connected with this expression. In other words, a clear distinction should be made between 'text' (in inverted comas), as a certain unit of language expression, and what this unit refers to, what it represents in referential terms, what it means (that is to say what constitutes its 'content'), and what I shall be presenting by means of italicised *text*.

No meanings of a 'text', therefore no *text,* is included in the expression 'text'. However, the meanings of a 'text', as is the case with the meanings of 'words' and 'sentences', can be interpreted in various ways – either as some entities existing beyond this expression or as some pure functions of this expression. Still, in neither case is the meaning its inherent component – neither structural nor material, neither of 'text' nor 'word' nor 'sentence' (see F. Grucza 1993). The reality which 'texts' refer to (which they represent), and much the same 'sentences' or 'words' – as expressions, should be 'divided' at least into two areas: namely the area of denotata and the area of designata. Denotata are facts/mental objects – primarily conceptual projections of designata, theoretical constructs, figments of the imagination. In brief, a clear distinction should be made between 'text' and what it refers to, and moreover, between the two areas of its semantic references – the area of designata and the area of denotata.

Also, in reflections upon the expression 'text', one should differentiate between at least two areas. In a particular case this expression may refer to either (a) its purely lexical form (structure) or (b) the actual material creating this form (structure). I am not going to elaborate on this issue now since it does not seem relevant for the purposes of our discussion. With reference to it, I shall only state that 'text' forms (structures), in the case of a particular speaker/listener are mental objects (facts), i.e. objects existing in his/her mind as certain elements of his/her structural and operational knowledge. 'Particular text realizations' constitute externalized objects, that is to say, autonomous objects which normally take the form of sounds (phonic form), letters (graphic form), or sometimes touch (tactile form). Reflections on 'texts' viewed 'as particular expressions' differ from those on their mental (language, idiolectal) forms, therefore a distinction should be made between the structures of the former and the structures of the latter. Only 'particular expressions' can be called signals, and these are, *inter alia*, 'particular texts' but not their 'forms'.

The fact, that translation competence is something that exists (deeply embedded) in a particular brain, and, as such, not amenable to direct empirical observation, constitutes only the first part of the problem that anybody who attempts to describe (reconstruct) any type of this competence, is confronted with. The other part of the problem consists in translation competence not being, in any particular brain, clearly isolated, in the fact that there are no clearly marked boarders between particular translation properties and any other properties in the mind of a translator. This means that yet another question translation studies must explore is how, and if at all, the scope of a particular translation competence can be defined or, in other words, on what criteria we can base our decision regarding what should be included within the scope of the competence in question and what should not.

If, however, the reconstruction of translation competence, enabling a subject to translate texts, can only be achieved by means of analysis of real texts, then a question arises: how can it be done? The answer to that question is: (a) by means of cognitive intellectual deliberations and (b) with the aid of equipment-supported research expanding on and/or verifying them. Cognitive deliberations have been undertaken since the emergence of translation studies, therefore, I am not going to dwell on this method of cognition any longer here. As far as the other type of research is concerned, we should commence discussing it with the statement that the semantic scope of the expression 'equipment-based research' is of a three-fold character: narrower, broader and the broadest. The narrower semantic scope of this expression means exclusively the activity of using a particular tool to perform a defined measurement of the material being researched and/or to perform a defined action (activity) upon this material. The broader scope of the meaning of the expression 'equipment-based research' means devising (planning) to perform an activity that uses a specific tool to perform a defined measurement of the material being researched and/or to perform a defined (action) activity upon this material, and subsequently to use this tool to perform the devised measurement of the material being researched and/or to perform the devised action (activity) upon it. Within the broadest scope of the meaning of the expression 'equipment-based research', we must also include action that consists in drawing conclusions from the result/outcome of the measurement of the material being researched and/or from the results/outcome of performing a defined action (activity) upon this material. As can be seen, the broader and the broadest scopes of the meaning of the expression 'equipment-based research' also encompass the preparation and intellectual verification of the 'pure' activity of using the particular research equipment.

The above remarks point to the fact that, actually, our (intellectual) cognition is based on a fundamental assumption (belief) that with the aid of our cognitive skills, senses, and abilities to apply them, and languages and abilities to use them, people are able to arrive at some cognition. In general, this is an assumption that people possess specific epistemic abilities. Whereas the concept of equipment-based cognition is based on an assumption (belief) that aided by some equipment, we are able to arrive at cognition of something, which is not amenable to direct sensual observation. At the same time it should also be stressed that any research equipment constitutes an exclusively, more or less perfect, extension of our senses, of our epistemic abilities. That is probably why F. Grucza (1983: 59), when writing on the physical tools of scientific research, introduced a differentiation between 'senses' and the 'instruments supporting them'.

Equipment-based research aimed at the cognition of translation processes was/is/can be carried out with the use of: (i) acoustic filters, sonographs, spectrometers, (ii) kimography, laryngoscopy, roentgenography, kinoroentgenography, palatography, labiography, (iii) electromagnetic techniques: EEC (electroencephalography) and MEG (magnetoencephalography), (iv) hemodynamic techniques: PET (positron emission tomography) and fMRI (functional magnetic resonance imagining), (v) ET (eye-tracking).

Hydrodynamic methods, PET and fMRI scans are purely diagnostic methods that enable the optical imaging of the brain and/or its activity. The resulting data do not provide information on the functions of particular brain regions. This can be obtained, only to a limited degree, with the use of optical imaging methods detecting cerebral cortex activity and multi-electrode measurements detecting the activity of selected neurons – EEG, MEG, Firm, and SPECT (Single Photon Emission Computed Tomography). On the basis of conclusions derived from the research done so far, it is assumed that carrying out research combining various methods is most effective. To what degree this statement can be applicable in translation studies research remains to be seen.

Nevertheless, fMRI research concerning various issues related to the use of language, mainly to the production and comprehension of longer or shorter utterances, has recently gained in popularity (for more on this topic see J. I. Skipper/S. L. Small 2005, C. J. Price 2010). Still, making use of functional brain imaging with fMRI is subject to many limitations:

> Apart from the type of information these methods provide, they also differ in the degree of ecological validity that can be achieved. Methods from the neurosciences require extremely artificial experimental situations in which the subjects must not move, not even their eyes and mouths, because such body movements cause artefacts which distort the recordings reflecting the cerebral activities caused by the cognitive translation processes proper. As a consequence, fMRT lends itself more to the investigation of interpreting processes, which, in contrast to translation processes, do not involve eye movements because an auditory input can be provided. For example, in fMRT experiments involving simultaneous interpreting, the subjects have to perform the interpreting task by thinking to themselves in a tube without actually speaking, and all this in an extremely noisy environment. This is obviously not an authentic interpreting situation, although it may yield interesting data for research purposes for which ecological validity is not an issue. (S. Göpferich/R. Jääskeläinen 2009: 171).

Moreover, functional brain imaging with fMRI is still insufficiently precise, very difficult to interpret, and the resulting research data elicited with Firm allow the researcher to arrive solely at general conclusions regarding only the involvement of large structures.

3. Eye-tracking to translation competences

Eye-tracking has turned out be the most effective translation process research method. Let us add, that the scope of its applicability is relatively broad. Most technologically advanced and currently widely used equipment-supported research concerns: (i) biometric identification, i.e. method of human iris recognition, (ii) so-called neuromarketing, i.e. research into consumers' (cognitive) responses to advertisements and products, (iii) website ergonomics, (iv) aerospace and space medicine (for a closer overview of eye-tracking methods see A. Duchowski 2003, N. Wade/B. Tatler 2005, K. Holmqvist et al. 2011[3]).

Eye-tracking employment in translation studies research is, according to D. D. Salvucci (1999), an important cognitive method because:

3 See also http://www.amazon.com/The-Moving-Tablet-Eye-Movement/dp/0198566166

> Eye movements are extremely informative as a data source for analysis of human cognition. Perhaps the most important reason for their usefulness is that eye movements indicate, generally speaking, the focus of visual attention. Although visual attention can move independently from eye-gaze location, attention always precedes eye movements: attention shifts to the location of the next fixation before the eye executes a saccade to that location […]. Thus, at the very least, eye movements provide clues to where the visual attention focuses at approximately the same time.

As a discipline, translation studies has just begun to develop interest in the possibilities of the applicability of eye-tracking methodology in experimental research. This interest is based on the belief that eyeball movements are motivated by the mental (cognitive) processes happening in the subject's mind. Consequently, on the basis of the subject's eyeball movements, a reconstruction of these processes can be made, in other words, hypotheses regarding the mental processes taking place in her/his mind can be formulated (N. Pavlović/ K. T. H. Jensen 2009: 94):

> We are assuming that the observable, measurable data that can be gained from eye-tracking are indicators of unobservable cognitive processes happening in the subject's mind during the translation tasks. […] We are further more assuming that the data related to the subjects' focus on the source text (ST) section of the screen are indicators of ST processing (reading, comprehension), while those data related to the subjects' focus on the target text (TT) section of the screen are related to TT processing (production, revision).

D. Stephen and S. O'Brien (2010: 2)[4] share a similar attitude:

> The main assumption behind eye-tracking is the so-called 'eye-mind hypothesis' (Ball et al 2006), which assumes that when the eye focuses on an object (e.g. a word) the brain is engaged in some kind of cognitive processing of that word. In eye-tracking investigations of reading, researchers typically measure the number of 'fixations' and the duration of these fixations to gauge how difficult the reading process is.

Summing up, let us however reiterate it once more: equipment-based experimental research (including, without doubt, eye-tracking research) carried out within the confines of translation studies is, from the scientific point of view, relevant as much as it measurably contributes to the creation of new or verification of previously acquired scientific knowledge, as much as it contributes to the scientific cognition of the translation studies object.

Let us at this point also bring up other methodological limitations of eye-tracking research. Firstly, they stem from a lack of standardized parameters for fixations and saccades – most eye-tracker providers set the length of fixations

4 See also D. C. Richardson/M. J. Spivey 2004.

and saccades on their own (for the needs of their devices) which, as a consequence, leads to different research results and may lead to different interpretations of these results. Problems concerning data interpretation may likewise derive from the lack of standardized measurement of data analysis (see R. J. Jackob/K. S. Karn 2003). And finally, they may also be related to the limited possibilities of eye-tracking data visualization.

As correctly pointed out by K. Holmqvist et al. (2011) in the conclusions to their book (*Eye Tracking: A comprehensive guide to methods and measures*), which presents a thorough analysis of the issues that relate to eye-tracking measurement, the current status quo, with its variety and multitude of measuring methods, consequently leads to a lack of broader compatibility in outcome interpretation.

> In fact, many measures are specific to certain application fields, and only appear in their journals. Sometimes a measure is limited to a single PhD thesis, with little availability to the entire community of eye-tracking users. The fact that eye-tracking publications are so fragmented make it very difficult to find the best methods and measures. […]
> Thus, somewhat paradoxically, despite there being a multitude of measures, many researchers do not find the ones that are relevant to them-sometimes it is not even apparent that a measure is relevant even when it is found. […] Finding the right measure is often the most difficult thing when designing an experiment, particularly for someone who is not trained in mathematics, computer science, or experimental psychology, or who is working outside established eye-tracking paradigms (K. Holmqvist et al. 2011: 455).

The authors' call to standardize software programmes, measurement methods and methods for data filtering, etc. should receive our support:

> Part of the problem is that no dedicated and widely known journals exist for eye-movement methodology (as opposed to theoretical journals). No one performs benchmarking tests of eye-tracker hard- and software systems, and no standardization committees exist for hardware and data quality measurements. There is a need for systematic evaluation of the programming routines developed by the providers of eye-tracking systems: methods for filtering, detecting, and calculating fixations, saccades, and other events should be agreed upon in the industry, in collaboration with researchers. Precise operational definitions for each measure should be standardized and stated in software manuals and help functions (*ibid.*).

4. Conclusions

Finally, when undertaking eye-tracking research, one should bear in mind not only the cognitive limitations of this method of imaging, but also the risks of succumbing to the temptation to interpret the acquired data in too simplistic a way.

The latter issue was lucidly brought up by A. Bojko and K. A. Adamczyk in their paper entitled *'Top misconceptions about eye-tracking'*. Although the authors' analysis specifically concerns how eye-tracking is incorporated into marketing research, their observations can be applied to the field of linguistics and translation studies with ease. Commencing their argumentation, the authors state:

> Eye-tracking is no longer a novel addition to the user experience (UX) research toolbox, used by only a few specialists. As more UX professionals incorporate eye-tracking into their studies, many misconceptions are being created and perpetuated. These false beliefs and questionable practices have given eye-tracking an undeserved bad reputation. It is time to start the process of change (p. 1).

The ten main misconceptions referring to both eye-tracking application and the interpretation of data acquired by means of this method, formulated by A. Bojko and K. A. Adamczyk in the above mentioned work, may also be applied to our field of studies. Let me quote them *in extenso* below:

1. All usability research can benefit from eye-tracking.
2. Eye-tracking is all about heatmaps.
3. Eye-tracking results are easy to interpret.
4. There is only one way to look at something.
5. Let's track and see what comes out!
6. There is a magic sample size for all eye-tracking user experience studies.
7. Eye-movement analysis can be done by watching gaze videos in real time.
8. The dot indicates exactly where a person looked and what they saw.
9. All data collected should be analyzed.
10. Anyone can do eye-tracking.

The above remarks lead us naturally to the most essential question to be answered by any researcher attempting an eye-tracking experiment: 'Heat maps, gaze plots . . . and what next'?

References

Ball Linden, J./ N. Eger/ R. Stevens/ J. Dodd (2006): *Applying the post–experience eye-tracked protocol (PEEP) method in usability testing*. In: Interfaces. 67. 15–19.

Benedetti, G./ G. Marchetti/ A. A. Fingelkurts (2009): *Mind Operational Semantics and Brain Operational Architectonics: a Putative Correspondence*. [http://www.ncbi.nlm.nih.gov/pmc/articles/ PMC2948146, accessed 12 December 2012]

Bojko, A./ K. A. Adamczyk (2010): *Top Ten Misconceptions about Eye-tracking*. In: User Experience. Volume 9, Issue 3, 3rd Quarter 2010 [http://www.usercentric.com/sites/usercentrc.com/files/Top%20Ten%20Misconceptions%20about%20ET%20%28UX%20Magazine%209.3%29.pdf, accessed 12 December 2012].

Croft, W. (1998): *Linguistic evidence and mental representations*. In: Cognitive Linguistics. 9(2). 151–173.

Dragsted, B./ G. Hansen (2009): *Exploring Translation and Interpreting Hybrids. The Case of Sight Translation*. In: Meta: journal des traducteurs / Meta: Translators' Journal. Vol. 54, Nr. 3, septembre 2009. 588–604. [http://www.erudit.org/revue/meta/2009/v54/n3/038317ar.pdf, accessed 12 December 2012]

Duchowski, A. (2003): *Eye-tracking Methodology. Theory and Practice*. London.

Göpferich, S./ R. Jääskeläinen (2009): *Process research into the development of translation competence: Where are we, and where do we need to go?* In: Across Languages and Cultures. 10 (2). 169–191. [http://www.akademiai.com/content/vp3x10p151ru10g8/fulltext.pdf, accessed 12 December 2012]

Göpferich, S./ A. L. Jakobsen/ I. M. Mees (eds) (2008): *Looking at eyes. Eye-tracking studies of reading and translation processing*. Copenhagen.

Grucza, F. (1981): *Zagadnienia translatoryki*. In: F. Grucza (ed.), Glottodydaktyka a translatoryka. Warszawa. 9–30.

Grucza, F. (1983): *Zagadnienia metalingwistyki. Lingwistyka – jej przedmiot, lingwistyka stosowana*. Warszawa.

Grucza, F. (1985): *Aspects of Translation and Translation Theory*. In: Kwartalnik Neofilologiczny. XXXII. 3/ 1985. 259–276.

Grucza, F. (1986): *Tłumaczenie, teoria tłumaczeń, translatoryka*. In: F. Grucza (ed.), Problemy translatoryki i dydaktyki translatorycznej. Warszawa. 9–27.

Grucza, F. (1990): *Zum Forschungsgegenstand und -ziel der Übersetzungswissenschaft*. In: R. Arntz/ G. Thome (eds), Übersetzungswissenschaft: Ergebnisse und Perspektiven. Tübingen. 9–18.

Grucza, F. (1993): *Interkulturelle Translationskompetenz – ihre Struktur und Natur*. In: A. P. Frank/ F. Paul/ H. Turk/ K.-J. Maaß (eds), Übersetzen verstehen, Brücken Bauen. Geisteswissenschaftliches und Literarisches Übersetzen im internationalen. Berlin. 158–171.

Grucza, F. (2008): *Germanistische Translatorik – ihr Gegenstand und ihre Aufgaben*. In: F. Grucza/ M. Olpińska/ H.-J. Schwenk (eds), Translatorik in Forschung und Lehre der Germanistik. Warszawa. 27–49.

Grucza, S. (2007): *Od lingwistyki tekstu do lingwistyki tekstu specjalistycznego*. Warszawa.

Grucza, S. (2008): *Instrumentalisierung von (Fach)Texten in der Ausbildung von (Fach)Übersetzern und (Fach)Dolmetschern – Grundannahmen*. In: I. Bartoszewicz/ J. Szczęk/ A. Tworek (eds), Fundamenta linguisticae. Wrocław/ Dresden. 299–310.

Grucza, S. (2010): *Język a poznanie – kilka uwag na temat rozważania ich wzajemnych relacji*. In: S. Grucza/ A. Marchwiński/ M. Płużyczka (eds), Translatoryka. Koncepcje – Modele – Analizy. Warszawa. 54–67.

Grucza, S. (2011): *Lingwistyka antropocentryczna a badania okulograficzne*. In Lingwistyka Stosowana / Applied Linguistics / Angewandte Linguistik. 4. 149–162.

Grucza, S. (2012a): *The Investigation of Translation Competences and Translation Processes*. In: Vestnik MGLU (in press).

Grucza, S. (2012b): *Zum Begriff „didaktischer Text" in der Fachtranslationsdidaktik*. In: M. Olpińska-Szkiełko/ S. Grucza/ Z. Berdychowska/ J. Żmudzki (eds), Der Mensch und seine Sprachen. Frankfurt/ M. 254–271.

Grucza, S. (2012c): *Grundzüge der Anthropozentrischen Translatorik*. In: Linguistica Silesiana. An international journal of linguistic studies (in press).

Holmqvist, K./ M. Nystrom/ R. Andersson/ R. Dewhurst/ H. Jarodzka/ J. von de Weijer (2011): *Eye-tracking: A comprehensive guide to methods and measures*. Oxford.

Jacob, R. J./ K. S. Karn (2003): *Commentary on Section 4. Eye-tracking in Human–Computer Interaction and Usability Research: Ready to Deliver the Promises*. Elsevier. 573–607.

Kielar B. Z. (1994): *Kształtowanie się translatoryki w latach 1972–1992*. In: B. Z. Kielar/ L. Bartoszewicz/ J. Lewandowski (eds), Polska szkoła lingwistyki stosowanej. Warszawa. 45–60.

Kielar, B. Z. (1986): *O adekwatne ujęcie językowych właściwości tłumacza*. In: F. Grucza (ed.), Problemy translatoryki i dydaktyki translatorycznej. Warszawa. 29–38.

Kielar, B. Z. (1988): *Tłumaczenie i koncepcje translatoryczne*. Wrocław.

Kielar, B. Z. (2003): *Zarys translatoryki*. Warszawa.

Luria, A. R. (1974): *Language and Brain Towards the Basic Problems of Neurolinguistics* In: Brain and Language. 1. 1–14.

Marchwiński, A. (1992): *Kompetencja kulturowa a kompetencja translatorska. Implikacje dydaktyczne*. In: F. Grucza (ed.), Bilingwizm, bikulturyzm, implikacje glotto-dydaktyczne. Warszawa. 243–253.

Marchwiński, A. (1993): *Z problematyki dydaktyzacji tłumaczenia*. In F. Grucza (ed.), Przyczynki do teorii kształcenia nauczycieli języków obcych i tłumaczy w perspektywie wspólnej Europy. Warszawa. 133–138.

Pavlović, N./ K. T. H. Jensen (2009): *Eye-tracking translation directionality*. In: A. Pym/ A. Perekrestenko (eds), Translation Research Projects 2, Tarragona: Intercultural Studies Group, 93–109 [http:/ / ebookbrowse.com/ eye-tracking-translation-directionality-pdf-d402604054, accessed 12 December 2012].

Płońska, D./ B. Bokus (2010): *Advanced Translation Strategies Exclusively for Professionals? Results of a Process–Oriented Translation Study*. In: B. Bokus (ed.), Studies in the Psychology of Language and Communication. Warszawa. 227–248.

Płużyczka, M. (2008): *Psycholingwistyczne aspekty dydaktyki translacji tekstów specjalistycznych (na materiale rosyjskich tekstów prawnych)*. University of Warsaw (unpublished PhD. Thesis).

Płużyczka, M. (2011a): *Eye-Tracking Analysen in der Translationswissenschaft. Zum Stand der Forschung*. In Kwartalnik Neofilologiczny. LVIII. 4/ 2011. 473–484.

Płużyczka, M. (2011b): *Okulograficzne wsparcie badań nad procesem tłumaczenia a vista*. In: Lingwistyka Stosowana/ Applied Linguistics/ Angewandte Linguistik. 4. 180–189.

Płużyczka, M. (2012a): *Eye-tracking Support of Translation Processes Analysis*. In: Vestnik MGLU (in press).

Płużyczka, M. (2012b): *Na co patrzy, a co widzi tłumacz a vista? Okulograficzne pytania translatoryki*. In: Lingwistyka Stosowana/ Applied Linguistics/ Angewandte Linguistik. 5. 65–74.

Price, C. J. (2010): *The anatomy of language: a review of 100 fMRI studies published in 2009*. In: Annals of the N.Y. Academy of Sciences 1191 (2010). 62–88. [http://qibawiki.rsna.org/images/5/5c/DrMohamed-Price_etal_2010-20100420.pdf, accessed 12 December 2012]

Richardson, D. C./ M. J. Spivey (2004): *Part 1: Eye–Tracking: Characteristics and Methods; Part 2: Eye-Tracking: Research Areas and Applications*. In: Encyclopedia of Biomaterials and Biomedical Engineering ed. G. Wnek/ G. Bowlin.

Salvucci, D. D. (1999): *Mapping Eye Movements to Cognitive Processes*. Doctoral Dissertation, Department of Computer Science, Carnegie Mellon University. [https://www.cs.drexel.edu/~salvucci/publications/TH99/Salvucci-TH99.pdf, accessed 12 December 2012]

Sandra, D. (1998): *What linguists can and can't tell you about the human mind: A reply to Croft*. In: Cognitive Linguistics. 9(4). 361–378.

Skipper, J. I./ S. L. Small (2005): *fMRI studies of language*. In: K. Brown (ed.), The Encyclopedia of Language & Linguistics: 2nd Edition. Oxford (Elsevier Science).

Stephen, D./ S. O'Brien, (2010): *Can MT Output be Evaluated Through Eye-tracking?* In: Machine Translation. 24(7). 1–13. [http://www.cngl.ie/drupal/sites/default/files/papers2/MTS-2009-Doherty.pdf, accessed 12 December 2012]

Toury, G. (1982): *A Rationale for Descriptive Translation Studies*. In: Dispositio. 7. 23–39.

Wade, N./ B. Tatler (2005 http://www.amazon.com/The-Moving-Tablet-Eye-Movement/dp/0198566166): *The Moving Tablet of the Eye': The Origins of Modern Eye Movement Research*. Oxford.

Problems, Objectives and Challenges of the Polish Translation Studies and Theory

Jerzy Żmudzki (Maria Curie-Skłodowska University in Lublin)

The above title contains, admittedly in a synthetic and announcing form, the most important goals of this paper; however, for its communicative efficiency, it is essential to elaborate on them in detail in the introductory part. The notions mentioned here will be instrumentally used as a vital frame of reference which will allow for compiling a general, necessarily selective and, I hope, valid characterisation of the theory of translation in Poland. I do not use the term 'Polish theory of translation' deliberately, since in my view of the mentioned reality along with its proper interpretation (and this is not only my opinion), such a phase in the development of the discipline discussed here has not been reached yet, which I will try to point out; this may, however, actually occur by the way of the necessary integration of the discipline with the indispensable participation of the recently reactivated Polish Association of Applied Linguistics. Therefore, I have great expectations of it, and, as one may judge by the number of the participants of this general meeting, I am not alone in this belief.

Nevertheless, before I proceed with providing a more detailed and, due to apparent constraints, also selective description of the problems relating to, *inter alia*, the integration degree of the theory of translation as a discipline as well as the reasons for such a state, let me first discuss certain distinguishable phases of the intricate development of the theory of translation, obviously starting with the presentation of certain facts constituting a genesis of its own. Being obligated by the potency of these facts, I will allow myself to adopt specific theoretical models of the theory of translation understood as a discipline that were principally developed by F. Grucza in a continuous sequence of their evolutionary modifications, as well as developed further by the continuators of this idea. These shall constitute a fundamental structural basis and a substantial comparative reference framework for my disquisitions.

The publishing of O. Wojtasiewicz's work *Wstęp do teorii tłumaczenia* (An Introduction to the *Theory of Translation*) in 1957 has universally been recognised as a significant moment of the establishment of the theory of translation in Poland by most active researchers in this field. Theoretical foundations presented therein have lost none of their interpretational relevance to this very day; moreover, they also have opened up paradigmatically significant vistas and directions in research and development of this discipline.

This is how they are evaluated in the works by, *inter alia*, F. Grucza (2007: 323), T. P. Krzeszowski (1992: 3) and T. Tomaszkiewicz (2008: 313–314).

Nonetheless, it is a series of works authored by F. Grucza since 1977 up until now that we owe the emergence of the proper conception of the theory of translation as a discipline. In particular, his work published in 1981 contains a thorough description of the main model of the *Translation Model* in terms of a *Communication Model* which is a point of departure for the description and explication of the translational reality, which as a result of the development of this discipline has grown into the fundamental object of investigation and thanks to its interpretive augmentation by B. Z. Kielar (1988) is known under the label *Translation Model.* As it is already well known, in the centre of this model stands a human-translator functioning as a subject in the network of relations with other natural objects of the system. Such a configuration allows for a clear-cut distinction and delineation of the autonomy of this new discipline due to the specificity of its main subject of investigation as well as the other objects. It is exactly the description of the specific features of individual objects, with an absolute predominance of the primary and central object which is the mentioned subject of translational actions and operations, that has become the fundamental research programme setting directions and a basic scope of interests within the field of study that is the theory of translation. The processes and people defined by the mentioned model of relationships have been recognised to constitute its autonomous subject, which simultaneously testifies to the autonomy of the theory of translation, whereas particular translational acts performed by particular translators and the effects of these actions have always constituted its research material. In his further elaboration of the foundations of this theory, F. Grucza (1990: 12–15) has made a distinction between two variants of the theory of translation: the *pure* and *applied* theory of translation. The task of the former is to generate descriptive-explicative knowledge, whereas the latter should generate applicative knowledge. Such a division gives rise to *de facto* two interpretational dimensions of translational reality whose characteristics is best rendered by the following questions:

A. Pure theory of translation:

1. Questions regarding the properties of the objects:
a) What is the nature of the objects of investigation?
b) What are these objects?
c) What are their constitutive and distinctive features?
d) How do these objects behave?
2. Questions regarding the functioning of the objects:
e) Why do these objects behave in such a manner and not otherwise?
f) What determines their specific functioning?

B. Applied theory of translation:

a) How can you influence a specific kind and manner of the behaviour of the objects or how can you manipulate them?

b) How can you change specific features of the objects?

c) How can you induce the ability of the objects to function in a desired way, and how can you generate their programmed competence?

In the context of these questions, while the theory of translation was undergoing the process of its constitution, the most important objective of the discipline was formulated. It consisted in reconstructing the system of rules underlying the translational competence of particular people that are able to effectively perform specific translational operations and actions in the realm of their psycholinguistic reality. Among other things, in this way it was possible to make a clear-cut and unequivocal separation of the theory of translation from *translation linguistics* (or *linguistic theory of translation*), which was practiced particularly until the 1990s at the Karl Marx University in Leipzig (GDR) but also in Poland, influenced substantially by contrastive linguistics. The research interest of translation linguistics was centred primarily on the intertextual-interlingual relations between the source text and the target text, which in practice was tantamount to the traditional study of the phenomenon of equivalence within the scope of systemic equivalence reconstruction. On the other hand, the definition and classification of the equivalence between the source and target text was dependent, to a great extent, on the adopted linguistic model of text interpretation. As a result of defining the objective of the theory of translation and its situating in the realm of the translator's psycholinguistic reality, combined with the progressive, further broadening of the notion of translational competence to include the cultural-communicative aspect, the notions of intercultural and transcultural translational competence appeared (F. Grucza 1993: 168–169). It meant, both in theory and praxis, that the dominant paradigmatic claims of the traditional translation studies, which were based on the system of categories specific to literary studies that involved also traditional and, to some extent, structuralist text comprehension, were definitely dismissed. In consequence, the theory of translation dissociated itself from translation studies that were exclusively literature-oriented.

Another element differentiating the theory of translation from traditional translation studies and, at the same time, complementary to the translational model and its essential feature, was communicative interactivity of all active communication participants in the process of translation. In a desiderative sense, F. Grucza (*ibid.* 161) argues that an equally important objective of the theory of translation is to access the specific mental spaces of other participants of translational model, besides the translator's very own, as well as to describe their specific properties in the mentioned area of their activity. Upon following this line of holistically oriented global and communicative interpretation as well as upon applying consistently the categories introduced principally by German text linguistics, in several of my works (J. Żmudzki 2005, 2006, 2008a, 2008b, 2008c, 2009), I have granted myself the freedom to introduce the category of a translation *task* (also understood as a communication task) to the translational model understood in terms of a certain kind of a communicative model. Through this interpretative and, at the same time, modelling intervention, the translational model gains, adequately to its reality, strategic and communicative dynamics. Hence, the postulated holism of the concept of the theory of translation is further broadened (F. Grucza 1996: 42) to encompass 'the translation of every possible kind of human expressions, but primarily the so-called para- and extra-linguistic expressions (thus far attributed mainly to culture, but not to communication media)'.

In this way, through defining its capacity, the holistic formula of the theory of translation is given the status of an integration theory and, at the same time, allows for different kinds of translation including inter- and intralingual, interlectal and intersemiotic, and further both the literary and non-literary texts to be included in its object set. Those texts are interpreted, transformed in the process of translation and appropriately produced by competent translators depending on communicative situation, translation type, and a strategically determined mode of transfer within the area of cognitive profiling which is performed in the translator's mind.

In consequence, in its complex specificity this set includes also different kinds of translators existing in strict correlation with functionally determined scope and kind of translator's competence. Other subsets consist of different types and kinds of communication and translation, different types and kinds of texts, as well as different strategically determined methods of transforming source texts into target texts, thanks to which they become functional tools of efficient communication with target recipients.

Another, for the theory of translation evolutionarily significant aspect of the mentioned holistic formula constitutes a constant level of its receptive sensitivity to the theoretical broadening of research perspective through the appropriate implementation of new interpretational paradigms from other disciplines, and from broadly understood linguistics in particular. And thus, using the diagnosis formulated by E. Łabno-Falęcka (1995) with regard to determining which translation theories played the dominant role in the development of the theory of translation (in Poland), it can be acknowledged that they can be recognised in the conception of the theory of translation practised and further developed primarily by a huge team of researchers and academic teachers of the Institute of Applied Linguistics at the University of Warsaw. Following the author cited above, these dominant translation theories that have also influenced the theory of translation in Poland include: 1. descriptive-functional theory, 2. prescriptive-functional theory, 3. linguistic- and literary-oriented integration theory of translation in two variants: a) transdisciplinary, based on the theory of linguistic acts, and b) communicative-cognitive. All of them have received proper development, elaboration and application in studies and works by the aforementioned team and institute and have been described in a number of publications by B. Z. Kielar, in particular, in her article from 1996 entitled *Kierunki rozwoju translatoryki w okresie 1970–1995* (The development directions of the theory of translation 1970–1995), in the book by D. Urbanek (2004) *Pęknięte lustro. Tendencje w teorii i praktyce przekładu na tle myśli humanistycznej* (Broken Mirror. Tendencies in translation theory and practice against the background of humanistic thought), and further in the collective work by B. Z. Kielar/L. Bartosiewicz/J. Lewandowski (1994) *Polska szkoła lingwistyki stosowanej* (The Polish School of Applied Linguistics), as well as in numerous bibliographic-annalistic publications by J. Lewandowski.

While within the Institute of Applied Linguistics, the Department of Specialized Languages or the whole Faculty of Applied Linguistics at University of Warsaw in its present form the theory of translation as outlined above could be 'cultivated', to certain degree, in the whole extension of its internal diversity as a discipline and, simultaneously, exist thanks to such forms of institutionalisation as an idealisation *sui generis* through, probably, the highest level of integration, on a national university scale this landscape appeared and appears to be divided and diverse in the sense of profiling the conception of this discipline, and hence also its research paradigms.

The dominance of the aforementioned theories very clearly characterises individual academic research centres. And thus, the descriptive-functional theory deriving from G. Toury's conception of 'Descriptive Translation Studies' and 'Translation Studies' is represented, *inter alia*, by the German studies under the lead of M. Krzysztofiak of Adam Mickiewicz University in Poznań. Her research interest (M. Krzysztofiak 1999) centres on the function of literary translation in the target culture polysystem and the relationship between a translation and the horizon of target culture expectations, as well as the analysis of the individual relationship between each translation and the source text understood as a unique and one-time creation due to the fact that each literary work is both individually and creatively understood and interpreted. M. Krzysztofiak recognises the methodology adopted by literary studies to be fundamental for the study of literary text translations, but also other translation types. In a, to some extent, separatist way she postulates bringing to life the theory of translation that is exclusively linguistics-oriented on the one hand, while on the other she advances the creation of *translatology* whose main objective would be to study literary texts. The rationale for putting forward such a division, which arises from the heterogeneity of texts, would be acceptable if, due to the impetus for pragmatic claims, the so-called pragmatic translation, i.e. non-literary text translation, was not subsumed under translatology as well.

The prescriptive-functional method and theory, known also as *skopos theory* postulated by K. Reiss and H.-J. Vermeer, can be found in the works by Z. Berdychowska, Z. Weigt, R. Szubert and partially in my own works and works by others representing and practising the translation of specialised texts (S. Grucza 2008, 2012a), both in theory and practice, and affiliated with Jagiellonian University in Kraków, University of Lodz, University of Silesia in Katowice, University of Wrocław, University of Gdańsk, and of course, Institute of Applied Linguistics and Institute of Anthropocentric Linguistics and Culturology at University of Warsaw represented by B. Z. Kielar, S. Grucza, A. Marchwiński, M. Płużyczka, and others, as well as Institute of Applied Linguistics at A. Mickiewicz University. The characteristic feature of this movement is a prospective target text (*translatum*) orientation and bringing into focus the category of the aim, or purpose of a translation and the action of translating. On this teleological perspective a text is subjected to specific mechanisms of deconstructive interpretation as a system of signs which only through the consideration of their situational embeddedness lose their multivalency. The text is (being) constructed only in the act of its reception that is strategically translation purpose-profiled.

The third group of theories together with the research methodology developed and applied by them incorporates a descriptive-explicative potential and a particular level of knowledge arising from text linguistics, pragma- and psycholinguistics, cognitive linguistics, literary studies and communication theory. The translation phenomena relating to the multidimensionality of text existence and functioning are investigated with use of appropriate tools. The transdisciplinary movement is best represented by Z. Wawrzyniak of the University of Rzeszów, renowned linguist and text specialist, expert in literature, poet and outstanding translator of poetry and thus a living epitome of theory and practice combined in one flesh. Because texts, according to Z. Warzyniak, have the status of transphenomena, i.e. they are at the same time cognitive processes and social products, they require a transdiciplinary approach understood as an integrated interpretational perspective generated by different scientific disciplines. Such an transdysciplinary and integegrated understanding of translation is postulated by Z. Wawrzyniak (2004 and 2006). The term integrist in the sense described above may also be attributed to K. Lipiński of Jagiellonian University and University of Rzeszów, Germanist, expert in literature, but also cognitivist and German poetry translator who, blessed with extraordinary talent and linguistic creativity, produces congenial translations. In Lipiński's view (2004: 120–135), in the process of translation a text is an instrument of communication, a complex material sign and, simultaneously, a message which on the one hand represents in a sign-manner the inner world of the author of the text, and on the other evokes the congruent and consensual mental-cognitive state of the recipient's inner world through a conventional or unconventional interpretation of this textual macro-sign. A similar cognitive perspective of research and literary text interpretation characterises the activity of E. Tabakowska representing English Studies at Jagiellonian University. She formulates her unique understanding of translation processes in many works, in particular in her publication from 2001 entitled *Językoznawstwo kognitywne a poetyka przekładu* (English version from 1993: *Cognitive Linguistics and Poetics of Translation*). A characteristic feature of her approach is the interpretational extraction of cognitive text profiles and thus the reconstruction of the cognitive inner world of a given author. A similar cognitive approach in the interpretation of translation phenomena represents T. Krzeszowski, Anglicist of University of Gdańsk. In his understanding of translation processes we can recognise significant references to the theories by Lakoff and Johnson as well as Langacker. Yet another, interesting variant of the integrational theories corresponding with K. Lipiński's model constitutes communicative-cognitive translation theory by K. Hejwowski (2004) representing Institute of Applied Linguistics at University of Warsaw. According to this theory, the task of a translator (of literary texts) is to provide a recipient with access to all interpretive trails, references and intertextuality indicated in a source text, because in this way the recipient is given the opportunity to understand and reconstruct to some extent the author's cognitive basis. In this way it is possible for communication to be established despite and beyond existing differences in culture-determined cognitive models of the world, both individual and collective. Since people do not perceive the world in the same way, communication including translation communication can only be and, in fact, it is approximate. However, already the cognitive approximation for the purpose of the explication of the world creates the basis for achieving the communicative goals and not only. In my works (2006 and 2009) I refer to this as the *collocution of the goals* of communication participants within the concept algorithm: co-operation, co-ordination and communication, which in consequence, through the introduction of the category of translation task constituting a specific strategic translation profile, allows for a more comprehensive consideration of the strategic aspect within a dynamic interpretation of the complex of translation actions. Of course, such modelling of translation reality is reminiscent of the theories by Krings, Lörscher and Kautz, all of which are based on the strategic conception of communication in general, and translational conception in particular, which is also realised as an element of the translation problem solution strategy. The conception of translation postulated by K. Hejwowski deserves attention for one more reason, namely because it introduces translation, though not radically yet, but still into the field or dimension of cultural discourse(s) which determine the perception and interpretation of the world. A certain kind of notional affinity may also be found in the works from 2006 by T. Tomaszkiewicz representing Romance studies.

A synthetical description of the above theories, even if not dominating then certainly distinguishable and exerting some paradigmatic influence, marks certain fields of research covering a great variety of topics that typify individual university centres scientifically and didactically interested in the theory of translation, according to their topics of preference and projects run by them. It has to be noted here that apart from Institute of Applied Linguistics and Institute of Anthropocentric Linguistics and Culturology at University of Warsaw extensive research in the field of consecutive interpreting is also conducted in, *inter alia*, Institute of Applied Linguistics at A. Mickiewicz University, Department of Applied Linguistics at Maria Curie-Skłodowska University in Lublin, UNESCO Chair at Jagiellonian University, University of Lodz. Other research projects concern simultaneous interpreting and are carried out at Jagiellonian University and partially in Department of Applied Linguistics at M. Curie-Skłodowska University and University of Lodz; research projects in the field of on-sight (a-vista) translation are continued in Department of Applied Linguistics at M. Curie-Skłodowska University; intercultural competence is investigated in Institute of Applied Linguistics A. Mickiewicz University. The broadest spectrum of research topics is covered by projects with different profiles encompassing the fields of specialised languages, specialised texts, specialised communication and specialised translation that are carried out, first and foremost, at the Department of Specialised Languages at University of Warsaw, in Institute of Applied Linguistics A. Mickiewicz University, Institute of German at: Jagiellonian University, University of Lodz, University of Silesia, University of Szczecin, University of Gdańsk. Presently the most popular thematic and research field constitutes the so-called audiovisual translation (T. Tomaszkiewicz 2006, A. Mickiewicz University, M. Curie-Skłodowska University) or media translation due to the expansion of media in mass communication. Certainly, it is the field of the highest cognitive appeal.

A further unquestionable research challenge poses situating respective projects in the area of discourses mentioned above and their influence on the course of relevant translational processes such as interpretation and cognitive transfer determined by a given translation or interpretation strategy. However, the greatest research challenge poses now the bioneural dimension of a human-translator that is functionally linked to the psycholinguistic dimension. The empirical investigation of the specific translational processes in the mental sphere of a translator is possible thanks to the equipment available in Polish medicine which allows for bioneural imaging, i.e. the visualisation of some unfolding neuronal processes. The result of applying these experimental tools is functional magnetic resonance imaging of the brain performing various tasks in its specific activity areas and in specialised centres. The dynamic broadening of research perspectives contributes directly to the increase in the variety of topics explored by the researchers, which is a universal phenomenon of the theory of translation not only in Poland. On the other hand, with reference to the general diagnosis of the development tendencies in the theory of translation made by T. Tomaszkiewicz (2008: 321), 'the variety of research topics obligates a translation theorist to refer to different linguistic and literary theories, but also to sociological, psychological, semiological, IT-related theories, etc.' (trans. RA) However, the most important reason for these multidisciplinary references is uncovering the multidimensional complexity of the research subject of the theory of translation.

The selective characteristic above may be seen to constitute development profiles of the theory of translation understood as the scientific discipline in Poland. Another type of a problem and phenomenon concerns the stages and forms of its institutionalisation and functioning in the field of respective research and translation didactics (S. Grucza 2004, 2005, 2012b, 2012c, M. Płużyczka 2009a, 2009b, 2009c, 2009d, 2011, 2013). This problem is connected with a specific phenomenon of the so-called *neophilological gravitation* of its consequence – which I will try to explain in the following. To start with, for the purpose of systematic transparency, two main and fundamental areas of institutional establishment of the theory of translation must be distinguished: first, within the world of science and university didactics including its different forms; and second, within the world of translatorial practice and relevant conditions underlying it. The theory of translation relating to the first area exists primarily as a component of applied linguistics established in appropriate forms of university structure including departments, chairs, institutes, or even faculties; secondly, as a part of neophilology having usually the form of an institute within the structure of a given university or college; and thirdly, in the institutionalised form of different so-called postgraduate studies in translation and interpreting. From historical perspective, the institutionalisation of the theory of translation is to be seen to first emerge in the development of the respective structures of University of Warsaw ; in particular, the first institution within University of Warsaw that included the theory of translation in the scope of its interests was the Department of Formal Linguistics led by O. Wojtasiewicz; another form of existence was provided by the College of Modern Languages under the auspices of University of Warsaw, but it was not actually established until after 1973 within the structure of Institute of Applied Linguistics in order to, as F. Grucza (2007: 324) describes, be able to continue its existence and development within the Faculty of Applied Linguistics at University of Warsaw (more on this can be found in respective publications by the scholars from Institute of Applied Linguistics). Yet another, to some extent, intermediate form of institutional establishment constituted the Department of Glottodidactics and Translatorics at A. Mickiewicz University, led first by W. Pfeiffer and then I. Prokop, which 4 years ago, led again by W. Pfeiffer, developed into the Institute of Applied Linguistics. Following the examples of these two institutes, but also others, more than 8 years ago the Department of Applied Linguistics was established in the Institute of German at M. Curie-Skłodowska University. This Department runs studies at two education levels and offers two vocational profiles: a teacher of two foreign languages and a translator/interpreter of two languages. Almost at the same time the following departments were established: Department of Applied Linguistics at University of Lodz or departments of translation studies in the Institute of English and Applied Linguistics at University of Lodz as well as at University of Rzeszów. In the university context the following should also be mentioned: the Centre for Translation Studies at University of Lodz, the School of Translation and Interpreting and Foreign Languages – now College of Modern Languages at A. Mickiewicz University, the College of Foreign Languages and Economy in Częstochowa as well as Studies for Translators and Interpreters at Jagiellonian University. In the last five years one can observe a sudden emergence of different 'applied linguistics' and 'translation studies', primarily at non-state universities, which constitute a separate and autonomous area of institutional higher education which I will not discuss here.

The second area of the institutionalisation of the theory of translation, especially in the period until the 1990s, constitute neophilology and foreign philology departments established within universities and subsequently also within non-state universities. At the outset of the 1980s, when the process of abandoning the classical formula of philology had just begun and the market demand for interlingual communication had gained increasing consideration, quite tentative attempts were made to gradually implement the theory of translation into the university programmes of neophilology education, principally as just a certain form of teaching translation as well as different and arbitrarily chosen theories of translation supporting it. Thus in the initial phase such translation didactics was nothing but enriched practical study of a given foreign language and most frequently it was present in the form of literary texts translation didactics. However, already in the 1990s we could observe the emergence of the departments or divisions of literary translation theory which educate and do research within this translation type. After 2000 a great programme expansion follows as a result of which translation or 'translatorial' specialisations are created with their ambitious objectives to primarily educate translators and compete with teaching specialisations, which was, and in fact had to be, included in the so-called 'graduate profile'. In particular, as a result of the introduction of 'New Matura Exam' and new legal regulations concerning higher education recruitment, as well as due to being aware of the threats of the approaching and more and more noticeable baby bust, strategies appeared in domestic universities which were aimed at competitiveness and candidate recruitment, *inter alia*, through establishing a translation specialisation on the neophilological studies all over the country. However, in many cases, and though up to this day, the declarations and aspirations did not fit in with the availability of proper staff, the level and kind of their competence, programme structure and its realisation, as well as the availability of didactically necessary media equipment. A very strange phenomenon was and still is the placement of such specialisation only on the first level of neophilological studies with reference to the specified graduate profile within this education scope which includes the amazing versatility of translator's skills. The awareness of real limitations and the verification of these conceptions by didactic reality imposes pressure on many institutes of neophilology to abandon these ideas or to resign now from running the full translation specialisation.

In the third area – postgraduate studies in translation and interpreting – the didactics of selected translation types dominates. This constitutes a form of professional specialisation that develops and completes neophilological studies. Such postgraduate studies are currently offered by University of Warsaw, A. Mickiewicz University, University of Wrocław, University of Lodz, Jagiellonian University and others.

A specific kind of institutionalisation of translation research studies are certain forms of their organisation and presentation involving a series of conferences and publishing series. Out of factual necessity and due to their significance I feel obliged to mention, first and foremost, the cyclic scientific conferences organised by Institute of Applied Linguistics at University of Warsaw that started in 1976 and continued with some small interludes up until today, where researchers could and can exchange scientific information, functionally bind specific research areas as well as create the awareness of autonomy of this discipline and, at the same time, its gradual integration. Another important and continued series of conferences devoted to translation research is *International Maastricht-Łódź Duo Colloquium on Translation and Meaning*. It is a series of scientific events organised since 1990 by the Department of Translation and Interpreting of Zuyd University in Maastricht and the Faculty of Philology of University of Lodz, and to be precise, by the the institutes of English, German and Romance Studies with the leading participation of B. Lewandowska-Tomaszczyk, M. Thelen, Z. Weigt and J. Sypnicki. Further conferences and publishing series related to the theory of translation are the results of the activity of Cracow *Tertium* Society for the Promotion of Language Studies which has been actively operating for more than 10 years under the auspices and support of Jagiellonian University and, to be precise, the institutes of English, German and Romance Philology with the active participation and support of E. Tabakowska, U. Dąbska-Prokop, Z. Berdychowska and many others. Since 2005 'Rocznik Przekładoznawczy' has been published, devoted to the study of translation theory, practice and didactics, edited by Lech Zieliński and Maciej Pławski representing Nicolaus Copernicus University. The aim of the editors of this periodical was to establish a discussion platform for the nationwide 'dialogue beyond the strict divisions into distinct philologies and neophilologies'. Since 2009 'Lingwistyka Stosowana/Applied Linguitics/Angewandte Linguistik' has been published, founded and edited by Sambor Grucza at the Department of Applied Linguistics at the University of Warsaw. Texts published in this journal concern various areas of applied linguistics, *inter alia*, translation studies. In fact, a great number of articles and reviews delivered by Polish and international authors is devoted to the translation theory and practice both in Poland and worldwide.

While the institutions and journals mentioned above create frames of reference for the organisation and coordination of the activities of the world of translation science, it is also worth taking note of such organisations as TEPIS (Polish Society of Sworn and Specialised Translators) and STP (Association of Polish Translators and Interpreters) which constitute institutionalised forms that unite the world of translation practice and conduct different forms of trainings, workshops and lectures devoted to principally practical issues also relating to translation job market and all its current operational modalities.

The institutional diversity of the theory of translation outlined here which arises directly from the local specificity of given neophilological studies is characterised by yet another kind of determinants of the shape and scope of this discipline, which for the purpose of this lecture I defined earlier as the phenomenon (or even the principle) of *neophilological gravitation* diversifying the theory of translation within the scope of individual neophilologies. This is a connotationally lighter version of the metaphor used by the Germanists' communities, following H. Orłowski (1987) and F. Grucza (1998, 2006, 2008), in order to conceptually capture the specificity of the conditions of each neophilology as a foreign philology in relation to the philology of the native language. Based on the natural entrenchment of each neophilology in the language, culture and land of a given foreign language on the one hand, and in the native language, culture (e.g. Polish culture) and land on the other, F. Grucza (1998 and 2006) formulated the theory explaining the autonomy of each neophilology as a foreign philology practiced outside of the land of language ethnic origin against each philology of the native language practiced in the land and environment of one's own national and ethnic origin, conditions and existence. During last year's Polish national conference organised by Polish Germanists' Society (Stowarzyszenie Germanistów Polskich/Verband Polnischer Germanisten) in Bronisławowo, which was devoted entirely to translation and the theory of translation, F. Grucza (2008) defined the specificity of the theory of translation that is determined by a given neophilology using a similar interpretation schema and pointing out the existence of double entrenchment ('double umbilical cord') also in the case of each theory of translation specific to a given neophilology. Owing to this entrenchment each of them has the so-called surplus relative to any philology practiced in the homeland in form of a certain area of translation didactics, research and practice. The phenomenon of natiolectal neophilological gravitation described above is nothing but upsetting the balance between the two entrenchments existing in reality in favour and direction of a given foreign philology, foreign language and all the worlds encapsulated in it, as well as gravitating towards them, which results in the situation where we have, for instance, the theory of translation that in its profile is specific exclusively to Romance, German, English or Russian philology etc. These theories of translation appear to be unilaterally oriented towards, for instance, the Romance philology in France, the English philology in the UK or USA, the German philology in Germany, the Russian philology in Russia etc. The tangible consequence of such a state is the narrowing of the receptive sensitivity of such theories of translation to the achievements of this discipline on the Polish nationwide scale within the scope of the general theory of translation and, as a result, the use of different names for designation of the very same discipline in the works relating to translation theory published in Polish; and thus, specialists in Romance studies will use the term *traductology*, specialists in English and Russian studies – *translation studies* or *translation theory*, for Germanists it will be *translatology* or *translation linguistics* etc. This attractive terminological diversity could even be accepted if only those names actually involved the practice of translation reflexion in its different aspects. A classic example of such unilateral, natio-philological understanding of the theory of translation provides the text by T. Tomaszkiewicz from 2008 dedicated to a very topical question: 'Where is the contemporary theory of translation heading?' In the very same article the author refers to the described discipline first as the theory of translation, then as traductology, further as translatology, translation studies etc., relating the whole area of operation of the contemporary theory of translation solely to the francophone area. Another consequence of this phenomenon is the use of typical notions relating to translation reality in their definitionally different, and sometimes even divergent senses. Evidence for that are provided very often at translation conferences encompassing different philological representations, where during scientific discussions it happens sometimes that someone breaks the proverbial 'open doors'. Thus a desired objective is to reach defintional consensus with regard to the fundamental notions categorising translation reality on the basis of the Polish nationwide institutionalised communication platform for this discipline. Otherwise, we may face a real threat of the hermetisation of certain areas of the translation discourse, and further even the rise of the phenomenon of neophilism.

The general characterisation of the theory of translation in Poland would not reach a complete description if translation didactics received no mention here, since apart from primary research area it constitutes an integral part of the theory of translation, thank to which this discipline is something more than just a certain area of applied linguistics. During the German studies-related event mentioned above and dedicated to the theory of translation F. Grucza once more identified the fundamentals of translation didactics, whose principle objective is to educate and train translators so that they can develop their specific competence understood as a mental property of specific persons in their specific cognitive environment. The full translator's competence, whose acquiring is the actual objective of academic training, includes translator's cognitive competence combined with practical translation competence. Certainly, it is not only a supplement to bilingual communicative competence, but it constitutes a significant added value, since every experienced translator has a set of self-generated and specific translation rules and skills constituting a certain added value, or a surplus of his/her skills and a certain added value, or else a surplus of knowledge as his/her so-called individual translation theory against any other monolingual communicative competence that is pre-translation-conditioned. Research in this area is centred on the identification and description of the factors constituting these added values, and thus it is concerned with persons and not (only) texts. Therefore research in this field is aimed at the reconstruction of the systems of principles and knowledge types underlying specific translational competences of individual translators and all this should be examined not only relative to a translation type, but also relative to a given language, its variants, technolects, and further text genres and types. Another important factor is the job market, its demands and needs which training and study programmes must take account of in order to provide their authenticity and professional adequacy. Reaching these goals and maintaining high education level is unattainable without the professional staff which absolutely excludes randomness and dilettantism. Only upon satisfying these conditions will translation graduates be able to, because they will have to, professionally meet the challenges posed by the translation job market. With regard to the institutionalised reality of translation didactics in Poland the above conditions are relatively best fulfilled by the curriculums and studies run within the university infrastructure including the institutes or departments of applied linguistics. Similar characteristics is attributable to postgraduate studies in translation and interpreting offered by some universities. In contrast, the largest deficits with reference to the foregoing requirements may be found in translation didactics offered as the so-called translation or translator's specialisation within university-based neophilological studies. Survey studies and interviews I conducted last year allow to give a diagnostic description of the current state of the translation theory in this institutionalised area:

1. The dominant translation type is translation of written texts and consecutive interpreting.
2. The presentation of relevant translation models and theories is marginalised or omitted.
3. Translation didactics is not based at all, or very generally at most, on macro-strategic models in the overall perspective of translation education. Defining only the final, even the most ambitious, goals is not enough. The practical intuition about the didactics concept and material selection is dominant.
4. In didactic reality the micro-strategy of a single text is usually practiced, mainly due to its linguistic and terminological attractiveness from teacher's perspective. The question of text types and their genological patterns remains an abstract notion of little cognitive availability and is processed didactically to the same extent.
5. Individual skills are very seldom defined in terms of the necessary competence components and the fulfilment conditions of specific translation types. As a result, they are not granted the status of transparent and micro-strategic goals of translation didactics. The reason for this is the lack of recognition of fundamental objectives and sense of didactic actions.

6. Even if the trained target competences are defined at a general level, their distribution between individual realisation stages that assumes and assures the desired progression in a particular order of developing specific skills does not gain necessary elaboration, nor does it come with the selection of appropriate didactic methods and techniques or exercises. Also with reference to the allotment of teaching time, semesters and hours we can observe extreme differences.
7. For these reasons, the participation in EU-programmes such as 'European Masters of Translation' is rather improbable or completely impossible.
8. An absolute rarity is the ability to provide professional translation traineeships coordinated and supervised by a professional academic teacher representing a given institute.
9. The closeness of professional practice imposes, in terms of improved translation quality, higher and higher demands with reference to implementing computer and Internet-based translation programmes integral to professional practice into translation didactics, to which demands neophilological translation didactics cannot face up.
10. A general problem remains still setting or defining a curricular frame of reference similarly to glottodidactics which would allow for the essential standardisation and optimisation of translation education in its different institutionalised forms, in particular in form of neophilological studies.

In addition to the area of translation didactics described in the foregoing and, to some extent, independently of it there exist legal acts that regulate and define the target ranges and levels of translator's competence required for the state exam certifying and admitting to practice as sworn translator. The exam is conducted by the special committee of experts appointed by the Ministry of Justice in accordance with the act of January 1, 2005 and the requirements stipulated in the Polish PN-EN 15038 standard: *Translation services – Service requirements*. Following A. Kubacki (www.kubart.pl), this standard defining translators' professional competences and applicable exclusively to written translation services differentiates between following essential competence types:

1. Translating competence comprises the ability to translate texts to the required level, in accordance with the requirements defined in the standard. In includes the ability to assess the problems of text comprehension and production as well as the ability to render the target text in accordance with the agreement concluded between the client and the translation service provider and to justify the results.
2. Linguistic and textual competence in the source language and the target language includes the ability to understand the source language and mastery

of the target language. Textual competence requires knowledge of text type conventions for as wide a range of standard-language and specialised texts as possible, and includes the ability to apply this knowledge when producing texts.

3. Research competence, information acquisition and processing include the ability to efficiently acquire the additional linguistic and specialised knowledge necessary to understand the source text and to produce the target text. Research competence also requires experience in the use of research tools and the ability to develop suitable strategies for the efficient use of the information sources available.
4. Cultural competence includes the ability to make use of information on the locale, behavioural standards and value systems that characterise the source and target cultures.
5. Technical competence comprises the abilities and skills required for the professional preparation and production of translations. This includes the ability to operate technical resources (as defined in the standard).

The standard also recommends that the competences described above should be acquired through at least one of the following ways:

a) formal higher education in translation (recognised degree),
b) equivalent qualification in any other subject plus a minimum of two years of documented experience in translating,
c) at least five years of documented professional experience in translating.

Due to this legal status the question about the possibility and extent of complying with these guidelines in the study curriculums designed for translators' education becomes very topical and justified, since it is the only institution conducting the certification mentioned. Which study curriculums can apply those guidelines? Is it possible at all? Should the instructions included in the documents cited above be seen as a minimal frame of reference for every studies of this type? On account of this, should each type of translation education lead to the achievement of proficiency level that would allow for obtaining professional qualifications? Is the problem of certification of any interest to universities or does it exist outside them and leave them unaffected?

Many answers to these and other questions can be found in the works by F. Grucza, K. Hejwowski, P. Płusa, J. Pieńkos, Z. Weigt, T. Gliwiński, and recently in a number of publications by J. Iluk and A. Kubacki. The problem of defining and even optimising these frames of reference is also raised during the conferences held at the Institute of German Philology of University of Wrocław.

The issues brought up here are the verbalisations of the remarks, fears and difficulties reported by the academic environment. They also reflect the specific state of involved awareness that can generate the desired activity thanks to the establishment of a new action platform whose foundation may certainly be the reactivated Polish Association of Applied Linguistics.

References

Berdychowska, Z. (1982): *Język fachowy w nauczaniu języka niemieckiego na studiach germanistycznych.* In: Germanica Wratislaviesia. XLIX. 59–64.

Berdychowska, Z. (1987): *Übungsgestaltung im fachübergreifenden Fremdsprachenunterricht auf der Grundlage von fachspezifischen Texten.* In: Skamandros – Germanistisches Jahrbuch – DDR – VR Polen. Warszawa. 152–159.

Berdychowska, Z. (1990): *Zum Stellenwert der Fachtextanalyse im Fremdsprachenunterricht.* In: W. Pfeiffer (ed.), Deutsch als Fachsprache in der Deutschlehrerausbildung in der Fortbildung. Poznań. 65–67.

Berdychowska, Z. (2001): *Zur Textsortenabhängigkeit der Personaldeixis in Fachtexten.* In: A. Kątny (ed.), Języki fachowe. Problemy dydaktyki i translacji. Olecko. 91–104.

Berdychowska, Z. (2002): *Redewiedergabe und der personaldeiktische Verweis.* In: D. Baudot (ed.), Redewiedergabe, Redeerwähnung: Formen und Funktionen des Zitierens und Reformulierens im Text. Tübingen.

Berdychowska, Z. (2004): *Ein Satz über den Diskurs.* In: F. Grucza/ M. Olpińska/ H.– J. Schwenk (eds), Konstrukte und Realität in der Sprach-, Literatur– und Kulturwissenschaft sowie in der Geschichtsforschung und Sozialwissenschaft. Warszawa. 108–119.

Berdychowska, Z. (2005): *Termin w przekładzie* (ed.), M. Piotrowska (ed.), Konteksty przekładowe. Język trzeciego tysiąclecia. III. Kraków. 119–129.

Berdychowska, Z. (2006): *Kontrastive Analysen von Fachtexten.* In: F. Grucza/ H.–J. Schwenk/ M. Olpinska (ed.), Texte Gegenstände germanistischer Forschung und Lehre. Warszawa. 293–300.

Dąbska–Prokop, U. (2005): *Język przekładu w oczach polskich przekładoznawców.* In: M. Piotrowska (ed.), Konteksty przekładowe. Język trzeciego tysiąclecia. III. Kraków. 183–197.

Grucza, F. (1981): *Zagadnienia translatoryki.* In: F. Grucza (ed.), Glottodydaktyka a translatoryka. Warszawa. 9–30.

Grucza, F. (1985): *Lingwistyka, lingwistyka stosowana, glottodydaktyka, translatoryka.* In: F. Grucza (ed.), Lingwistyka, glottodydaktyka, translatoryka. Warszawa. 19–44.

Grucza, F. (1990): *Zum Forschungsgegenstand und -ziel der Übersetzungswissenschaft.* In: R. Arntz/ G. Thome (eds), Übersetzungswissenschaft: Ergebnisse und Perspektiven. Festschrift für Wolfram Wilss zum 65. Geburtstag. Tübingen. 9–18.

Grucza, F. (1993): *Interkulturelle Translationskompetenz: ihre Struktur und Natur.* In: A. P. Frank/ K–J. Maaß/ F. Paul/ H. Turk (ed.), Übersetzen, verstehen, Brücken bauen. Geisteswissenschaftliches und literarisches Übersetzen im internationalen Kulturaustausch. Berlin. 158–171.

Grucza, F. (1996): *Wyodrębnienie się, stan aktualny i perspektywy świata translacji oraz translatoryki.* In: J. Snopek (ed.), Tłumaczenie: Rzemiosło i sztuka. Warszawa. 11–45.

Grucza, F. (1998): *Mitteleuropa – Deutsch – Auslandsgermanistik*. In: F. Grucza (ed.), Deutsch und Auslandsgermanistik in Mitteleuropa. Geschichte – Stand – Ausblicke. Warszawa. 27–44.

Grucza, F. (2006): *In– und Auslandsgermanistik: Zur Notwendigkeit ihrer Unterscheidung*. In: Deutsch als Fremdsprache. 43. 4/ 2006. 195–207.

Grucza, F. (2007): *Lingwistyka stosowana. Historia – zadania– osiągnięcia*. Warszawa.

Grucza, F. (2008): *Germanistische Translatorik – ihr Gegenstand und ihre Aufgaben*. In: F. Grucza (ed.), Translatorik in Forschung und Lehre der Germanistik. Warszawa. 27–53.

Grucza, S. (2003): *Badania z zakresu lingwistyki tekstu specjalistycznego w Polsce*. In: B. Z. Kielar/ S. Grucza (ed.), Lingwistyczna identyfikacja tekstów specjalistycznych. Warszawa. 35–55.

Grucza, S. (2004): *Od lingwistyki tekstu do lingwistyki tekstu specjalistycznego*. Warszawa.

Grucza, S. (2005): *Adaptacja tekstów specjalistycznych w dydaktyce przekładu*. In: M. Piotrowska (ed.), Konteksty przekładowe, Język trzeciego tysiąclecia. II. Kraków. 407–417.

Grucza, S. (2008): *Lingwistyka języków specjalistycznych*. Warszawa.

Grucza, S. (2012a): *Fachsprachenlinguistik*. Frankfurt/ M.

Grucza, S. (2012b): *Zum Begriff „didaktischer Text' in der Fachtranslationsdidaktik*. In: M. Olpińska-Szkiełko/ S. Grucza/ Z. Berdychowska/ J. Żmudzki (eds), Der Mensch und seine Sprachen. Frankfurt/ M. 254–271

Grucza, S. (2012c): *The Investigation of Translation Competences and Translation Processes* In: Vestnik MGLU (in press).

Heinemann, W./ D. Viehweger (1991): Textlinguistik. Eine Einführung. Tübingen.

Heinemann, M./ Heinemann W. (2002): Grundlagen der Textlinguistik. Tübingen.

Heinemann, W. (2005): *Textlinguistik vs. Diskurslinguistik*. In: M. Wierzbicka/ M. Sieradzka/ J. Homa (eds), Moderne deutsche Texte. Beirtäge der internationalen Germanistenkonferenz Rzeszów, 2004. Frankfurt/ M. 17–30.

Hejwowski, K. (2004): *Kognitywno komunikacyjna teoria przekładu*. Warszawa.

Iluk, J. (1998): *Problemy tłumaczenia nazw medycznych na przykładzie języka polskiego i niemieckiego*. In: Glottodidactica. XXVI. 123–136.

Iluk, J. (2000): *Problemy tłumaczenia nazw instytucji publicznych z języka polskiego na niemiecki i odwrotnie*. In: B. Z. Kielar/ T. P. Krzeszowski/ J. Lukszyn/ T. Namowicz (eds), Problemy komunikacji międzykulturowej. Warszawa. 193–213.

Iluk, J. (2008): *Zur Rechtfertigung des Übersetzens/ Übertragens im Fremdsprachenunterricht*. In: F. Grucza (ed.), Translatorik in Forschung und Lehre der Germanistik. Warszawa. 61–71.

Jurewicz, M. (2001): *Erklärungssequenzen in deutsch–polnischen Gesprächen. Eine Studie anhand konsekutiv gedolmetschter Texte*. Adam Mickiweicz University. Poznań (unpublished PhD Thesis).

Jurewicz, M. (2003): *Erklärungssequenzen in konsekutiv gedolmetschten Gesprächen*. In: Glottodidactica. XXIX. 5–23.

Kątny, A. (2001a): *Kontakty językowe a słownictwo specjalistyczne*. In: A. Kątny (ed.), Języki fachowe. Problemy dydaktyki i translacji. Olecko. 17–25.

Kątny, A. (ed.) (2001b): *Języki fachowe. Problemy dydaktyki i translacji*. Olecko.

Klonowicz, T. (1994): *Putting one's Heart into Simultaneous Interpretation.* In: S. Lambert, B. Moser-Mercer (ed.), Bridging the Gap: Empirical research in simultaneous interpretation. Amsterdam. 213–224.

Kielar, B. Z. (1981): *Nauczanie tłumaczenia w zakresie subjęzyka specjalistycznego.* In: F. Grucza (ed.), Glottodydaktyka a translatoryka. Warszawa. 111–125.

Kielar, B. Z. (1988): *Tłumaczenie i koncepcje translatoryczne.* Warszawa.

Kielar, B. Z. (1991): *Problemy tłumaczenia tekstów specjalistycznych.* In: F. Grucza: Teoretyczne podstawy terminologii. Wrocław/ Warszawa/ Kraków.

Kielar, B. Z. (1993): *Nauczanie tłumaczenia: rozważania nad ekwiwalencją i ekwiwalentnym tekstem przekładu.* In: F. Grucza (ed.), Przyczynki do teorii i metodyki kształcenia nauczycieli języków obcych i tłumaczy w perspektywie wspólnej Europy. Warszawa. 139–150.

Kielar, B. Z./ L. Bartoszewicz/ J. Lewandowski (eds) (1994): *Polska szkoła lingwistyki Stosowanej.* Warszawa.

Kielar, B. Z. (1996): *Kierunki rozwoju translatoryki w okresie 1970–1995.* In: Lingua Legis. 4. 20–27.

Kielar, B. Z. (2000): *O tłumaczeniu tekstów specjalistycznych.* In: B.Z. Kielar/ T. P. Krzeszowski/ J. Lukszyn/ T. Namowicz (eds), Problemy komunikacji międzykulturowej. Lingwistyka, glottodydaktyka, translatoryka. Warszawa. 235–248.

Kielar, B. Z. (2002): *Języki specjalistyczne a translatoryka.* In: J. Lewandowski (ed.), Języki specjalistyczne 2. Problemy technolingwistyki. Warszawa. 171–180.

Kielar, B. Z. (2003a): *TS w układzie międzynarodowej komunikacji zawodowej.* In: B. Z. Kielar/ S. Grucza (eds), *Lingwistyczna identyfikacja tekstów specjalistycznych.* Warszawa.

Kielar, B. Z. (2003b): *Zarys translatoryki.* Warszawa. 121–133.

Kopczyński, A. (1976): *Kilka uwag metodologicznych na temat studiów nad ustnym tłumaczeniem konsekutywnym.* In: F. Grucza (ed.), Lingwistyka stosowana i glottodydaktyka. Warszawa. 191–203.

Kopczyński, A. (1980): *Conference interpreting: some linguistic and communicative problems.* Poznań.

Koźbiał, J. (2003): *Übersetzungsforschung und Integration.* In: F. Grucza (ed.), Deutsch–polnische und gesamteuropäische Integration in Forschung, Lehre und Öffentlichkeitsarbeit der (polnischen) Germanistik. Warszawa. 361–366.

Krysztofiak, M. (1999): *Przekład literacki a translatologia.* Poznań.

Krzeszowski, T. (1988): *Wstęp.* In: G. Lakoff/ M. Jonson, Metafory w naszym życiu. Warszawa. 5–18.

Kubacki, A. (2004): *Niemieckie derywaty z* –ung *jako składnik grupy wyrazowej i ich odpowiedniki w języku polskim.* University of Silesia (unpublished PhD Thesis).

Lewandowski, J. (1992): *Informator: Instytut Lingwistyki Stosowanej 1972–1992.* Warszawa.

Lewandowski, J. (1994): *Scientystyczny model badań naukowych prowadzonych przez ILS w latach 1972–1992.* In: B.Z. Kielar/ L. Bartoszewicz/ J. Lewandowski (eds), *Polska szkoła lingwistyki Stosowanej.* Warszawa. 35–44.

Lewandowski, J. (1996): *Bibliografia przekładoznawstwa polskiego za lata 1955–1977.* In: Lingua Legis. 3.

Lipiński, K. (2004): *Mity przekładoznawstwa.* Kraków.

Łabno-Falęcka, E. (1995): *Phraseologie und Übersetzen.* Frankfurt/ M.

Małgorzewicz, A. (2003): *Prozessorientierte Dolmetschdidaktik.* Wrocław.

Marchwiński, J. (2003): *Determinanty ekwiwalencji przekładowej tekstów specjalistycznych.* In: B. Z. Kielar/ S. Grucza (eds), Lingwistyczna identyfikacja tekstów specjalistycznych. Warszawa. 147–158.

Olpińska, M. (2003): *Struktura podręcznika 'Tłumaczenie tekstów specjalistycznych'.* In: B. Z. Kielar/ S. Grucza (eds), Lingwistyczna identyfikacja tekstów specjalistycznych. Warszawa. 159–168.

Orłowski, H. (1987): *Die doppelte Nabelschnur fremdsprachlicher Germanistik.* In: A. Wierlacher (ed.), Perspektiven und Verfahren interkultureller Germanistik. München. 113–124.

Pisarska, A. I./ B. Tomaszkiewicz (1996): *Współczesne tendencje przekładoznawcze.* Poznań.

Płużyczka, M. (2009a): *Psycholingwistyczne aspekty dydaktyki translacji tekstów specjalistycznych.* University of Warsaw (unpublished PhD Theis).

Płużyczka, M. (2009b): *Ćwiczenia specjalistyczne w kształceniu tłumaczy – eksperyment badawczy.* In: Komunikacja Specjalistyczna. 2. 99–112.

Płużyczka, M. (2009c): *Dydaktyka translacji tekstów specjalistycznych – aspekt metodyczny.* In: A. Waszczuk-Zin (ed.), W kręgu problematyki technolektalnej. Warszawa. 285–312.

Płużyczka, M. (2009d): *Dydaktyka translacji – rozważania terminologiczne.* In: Przegląd Glottodydaktyczny. 26. 195–200.

Płużyczka, M. (2011): *Wybrane trudności translacyjne a proces translodydaktyczny.* In: S. Piotrowski (ed.), O nauczaniu i uczeniu się języka obcego dla potrzeb zawodowych. Lublin. 88–97.

Płużyczka, M. (2013): *Okulograficzne spojrzenie na trudności translacyjne.* In: Rocznik Przekładoznawczy. Studia nad teorią praktyką i dydaktyką przekładu (in press).

Reiss, K./ H.-J. Vermeer (1984, 1991): *Grundlegung einer allgemeinen Translationstheorie.* Tübingen.

Schatte, Cz. (2001): *Język reklamy a języki fachowe.* In: A. Kątny (ed.), Języki fachowe, problemy dydaktyki i translacji. Olecko. 71–79.

Szubert, R. (1998): *Zur Fachsprache der Juristik.* In: Orbis Linguarum. 8/ 1998. 139–146.

Szubert, R. (2004): *Wie verständigt man sich vor Gericht?* In: Kommunikation für Europa. Sprachkontakte–Sprachkulturen–Sprachenlernen. Szczecin. 165–171.

Szubert, R. (2008): *Rechtssprache als Gegenstand der Übersetzungsdidaktik.* In: F. Grucza (ed.), Translatorik in Forschung und Lehre der Germanistik. Warszawa. 222–238.

Tabakowska, E. (2001): Językoznawstwo kognitywne a poetyka przekładu. Kraków.

Tomaszkiewicz, T. (2006): *Przekład audiowizualny.* Warszawa.

Tomaszkiewicz, T. (2008): *Dokąd zmierza współczesna translatoryka?* In: K. Myczko/ B. Skowronek/ W. Zabrocki (eds), Perspektywy glottodydaktyki i językoznawstwa. Tom jubileuszowy z okazji 70. Urodzin Profesora Waldemara Pfeiffera. Poznań. 313–325.

Urbanek, D. (2004): *Pęknięte lustro: Tendencje w teorii i praktyce przekładu na tle myśli humanistycznej.* Warszawa.

Wawrzyniak, Z. (2002): *Zasady rozumienia jako warunki konstytutywne tłumaczenia.* In: J. Koźbiał (eds), Recepcja. Transfer. Przekład. Warszawa. 39–46.

Wawrzyniak, Z. (2004): *Textwissenschaft als Transdisziplin.* In: A. Dębski/ K. Lipiński (eds): Perspektiven der polnischen Germanistik in Sprach– und Literaturwisenschaft. Kraków. 325–333.

Wawrzyniak, Z. (2006): *Textbildungsprinzipien.* In: F. Grucza (eds), Texte Gegenstände germanistischer Forschung und Lehre. Warszawa. 31–41.

Weigt, Z. (2000): *Pragmatyczno–językowe aspekty powszechnej informacji medycznej na przykładzie polskich i niemieckich ulotek do lekarstw.* In: K. Michalewski (ed.), Regulacyjna funkcja tekstów. Łódź. 425–433.

Weigt, Z. (2001): *Języki fachowe w pragmatyce zajęć tłumaczeniowych.* In: A. Kątny (ed.), Języki fachowe, problemy dydaktyki i translacji. Olecko. 129–138.

Weigt Z. (2002a): *Ausgewählte Probleme bei der Interpretation und Übersetzung deutscher und polnischer Fachtexte.* In: B. Lewandowska-Tomaszczyk/ M. Thelen (eds), Translation and Meaning, 6. Maastricht. 395–401.

Weigt, Z. (2002b): *Fachkommunikative Komponenten im Übersetzungsunterricht für Germanistikstudenten.* In: W. Kalaga/ Z. Mielczarek/ T. Rachwał/ D. Pindel (eds), Literature and Linguistics. Literatur und Linguistik. 1. Reihe: Academic Papers of College of Foreign Languages. Wissenschaftliche Beiträge der Hochschule für Fremdsprachen. Częstochowa. 195–205.

Weigt, Z. (2004): *Język specjalistyczny – dydaktyka – słownik.* In: J. Lewandowski (ed.), Języki specjalistyczne 4. Leksykografia terminologiczna – teoria i praktyka. Warszawa. 202–212.

Weigt, Z. (2006): *Fachtexte als Gegenstand der Didaktik.* In: F. Grucza (ed.), Texte Gegenstände germanistischer Forschung und Lehre. Warszawa. 166–174.

Wille, L. (2001): *Język fachowy w dydaktyce translacji na przykładzie języka sportowego.* In: A. Kątny (ed.), Języki fachowe, problemy dydaktyki i translacji. Olecko. 39–150.

Wille, L. (2003): Semantische Figuren in der Übersetzung. Marburg.

Żmudzki J. (1998a): *Zum Stand der Translatorik in Polen.* In: F. Grucza (ed.), Deutsch und Auslandsgermanistik in Mitteleuropa. Geschichte – Stand – Ausblicke. Warszawa. 487 – 499.

Żmudzki, J. (1998b): *Konsekutivdolmetschen – Handlungen, Operationen, Strategien.* Paris etc.

Żmudzki, Jerzy (2004a): *Blattdolmetschen als eine bekannte und verkannte Sondersorte der Translation.* In: A. Dębski/ K. Lipiński (eds), Perspektiven der polnischen Germanistik in Sprach– und Literaturwissenschat. Kraków. 353–363.

Żmudzki, J. (2004b): *Translationsaufgabe als Kommunikationsaufgabe – Etablierung eines Kategorie–Begriffs.* In: I. Bartoszewicz/ M. Hałub/ A. Jurasz (eds), Werte und Wertungen. Sprach-, literatur- und kulturwissenschaftliche Skizzen und Stellungnahmen. Wrocław. 320–330.

Żmudzki, J. (2005a): *Transferprozesse und Typen beim Vollzug des Konsekutivdolmetschens.* In: G. Antos/ S. Wichter (eds), Transferwissenschaft. Wissenstransfer durch Sprache als gesellschaftliches Problem. Berlin etc. 251–264.

Żmudzki J. (2005b): *Ekspansja specjalistycznych tekstów docelowych w tłumaczeniu konsekutywnym.* In: M. Piotrowska (eds), Konteksty przekładowe. Język trzeciego tysiąclecia. III. Kraków. 349–358.

Żmudzki, J. (2006): *Texte als Gegenstände der translatorischen Forschung und Lehre.* In: F. Grucza (ed.), Texte Gegenstände germanistischer Forschung und Lehre. Warszawa. 41–61.

Żmudzki, J. (2007a): *Das Fremde in der Translation.* In: B. Maksymčuk/ H. Eggert/ I. von der Lühe (eds), Kulturräume und Erinnerungsorte aus sprach-, literatur- und kulturwissen-schaftlicher Sicht. Lwiw. 107–128.

Żmudzki, J. (2007b): *Translacja w dydaktyce języka obcego na przykładzie ćwiczeń tłumaczeniowych w polskich podręcznikach do nauki języka niemieckiego – próba odtabuizowania.* In: H. Kardela/ T. Zygmunt (eds), Rola językoznawstwa w metodyce nauczania języka obcego. Chełm. 25–35.

Żmudzki, J. (2008a): *Ein holistisches Modell des Konsekutivdolmetschens.* In: B. Lewandowska–Tomszczyk/ M. Thelen (eds), Translation and Meaning, 8. Maastricht, Łódź. 175–183.

Żmudzki, J. (2008b): *Intermedialität in der Translation.* In: K. Myczko/ B. Skowronek/ W. Zabrocki (eds), Perpektywy glottodydaktyki i językoznawstwa. Poznań. 333–345.

Żmudzki, J. (2008c): *Das Problem des Übersetzens im Deutschunterricht. Fortsetzung einer Diskussion.* In: J. Janoszczyk/ L. Krzysiak/ J. Żmudzki (eds), Deutsch lernen und Lehren mit Lehrwerken. Vergangenheit, Gegenwart, Zukunft. Lublin. 99–115.

Żmudzki, J. (2008d): *Translationsdidaktik in den polnischen Germanistikinstituten. Realität und Anspruch.* In: F. Grucza (eds), Translatorik in Forschung und Lehre der Germanistik. Warszawa. 71–96.

Żmudzki J. (2008e): *Zum Stand der Translationsdidaktik in den polnischen Germanistikinstituten. Ein Arbeitsbericht.* In: Glottodidactica. XXXVI. 153–172.

Żmudzki, J. (2009): *Text(e) in der Translationsperspektive – einige ausgewählte Aspekte.* In: M. Czyżewska/ W. Czachur (eds), *Od słowa do tekstu. Zmiana paradygmatów w językoznawstwie*. Warszawa. 39–45.

Knowledge – Transference – Translation

Marta Małachowicz (University of Warsaw)

Introduction

Considering the three concepts presented in the title, one can easily find relation between them all, with the middle one – transference as the linking notion for the other two. Transference sometimes seems to be perceived literally, especially when popularly understood, which probably results directly from expressions like 'to acquire knowledge', 'to spread knowledge'[1] etc. We want to underline in the very beginning that this literal way of understanding knowledge transference is wrong. In fact, knowledge is in no way transmitted. Nobody is able to acquire any piece of knowledge in literal sense. Actually, everybody has to create or reconstruct it on his/her own. If 'transmitting' knowledge was possible, some loss of it would be implied within this process. This kind of misunderstanding the process is due to inaccuracy of language expressions in representing certain meanings.

1. Knowledge

Discussion on the concept of *knowledge* is focused on two traditions, which sources date back to the ancient philosophy. One of them assumes that the real world has certain structure (hierarchy) that is perceived by human mind (sensory perception) and recreated by it on the basis of induction. The second tradition considers cognition conditional on personal experience of a human being that helps him/her to activate certain 'areas' of a cognitive system – in this case the human being in a way retrieves information that was given to him/her before (T. P. Krzeszowski 1997: 24–25).

In a long-running discussion on knowledge two different concepts are distinguished. These are *general knowledge* and *domain-specific knowledge*. General knowledge is understood as a particular state of mind based on the set of mental components which can be both genetically determined (inherited) and created ('acquired') through experience. These genetically inherited components are sometimes called natural knowledge or genetic knowledge. The components created by experience are, on the other hand, the result of socialization, education, independent acts of cognition or emotional experience of a human

1 In Polish expressions like 'przyswajanie wiedzy', 'przekazywanie wiedzy' or 'dostarczanie wiedzy' are commonly used.

being. Therefore, diverse activities and acts of cognition lead to creating knowledge of the reality, and the results of these acts and activities are expressed in the set of statements, propositions, hypotheses and theories. The other distinguished concept is domain-specific knowledge. It is defined as a kind of scientific knowledge that shares all its features, i.e. relativity, ability to be verified and time variability. Domain-specific knowledge of separate fields constitutes the body of scientific knowledge. Unlike general knowledge, domain-specific knowledge is not only theoretically and experimentally proved but in its very nature it is oriented at creating new facts in professional activity (NEP 2004; STP 2005).

Regardless of the presented division, it is important to emphasize that knowledge is the property of living creatures (human beings) and only in connection with them we can consider its existence. The question which organisms can be 'equipped' with knowledge leads to hypotheses and assumptions that have considerable ethical importance. For this issue, compare for example F. Grucza (1997: 12–13):

> 'All living organisms, especially those that have brains, are equipped with some knowledge. [...] It is not true that only people are given their natural knowledge, or only people inherit genetically determined ability of creating knowledge. Actually, even plants possess some knowledge. They 'know', after all, when, in what conditions, what season etc. they can, should or should not, for instance, sprout, come into leaf, blossom etc. Some knowledge is accumulated in every seed, fruit, and every potato and of course in every fertilized egg. [...] It has to be defined first what knowledge can be created, recreated or reconstructed only by human beings and then the question can be posed – what knowledge some living organisms are able to store.' (English translation by M. Małachowicz)

The human beings' distinctive feature is, among other things, knowledge of the language potential, i.e. their ability to comprehend and produce language and use it in a creative way. Knowledge of the language that exists in every human being's brain in the form of referents constitutes the basis for developing individual knowledge of the reality. The knowledge units like notions or concepts are represented in statements (material means of expression). Nevertheless, knowledge exists independently of the verbal form, it is quite sure that it has to exist prior to the verbal expression (see S. Grucza 2012a, 2012b, 2012c).

In the process of its evolution, scientific knowledge, when reaching a certain stage of development, requires an appropriate form of expression. There are two basic forms of presenting scientific knowledge. The first one is a code for knowledge recording in the form of symbols, statements and means of cohesion. The second one is a variety of specialist texts (secondary in relation to a sign).

Scientific language (as any other LSP) is, in most cases, a combination of artificial (in the sense of symbols and precisely defined terms) and natural languages. Therefore, LSP can be defined as a conventional semiotic system based on natural language that represents domain-specific knowledge (STP 2005).

In the stage of encoding (representing), scientific knowledge is confronted with completely different system, knowledge of the language system in a human brain. This system forms a hierarchical structure, the base of which are concepts and various relations between them. A word in every language constitutes inseparable whole with its meaning. Similarly, 'contents' of scientific knowledge become inseparable component of scientific language. Scientific knowledge represented through terminological units (terms) in a way gains new quality becoming the constituent of a certain LSP. This 'encoding of knowledge' is always connected with creating a text. Therefore, when contents of knowledge start to function as text semantics, scientific knowledge in qualitative sense gains a new form of existence.

Specialist texts give the possibility to represent domain-specific knowledge in a new form through modelling the systems of notions and the systems of terms. Step by step, according to general-to-specific pattern, relations in hierarchical structure of a certain field of knowledge are established. The stage of revealing fundamental logical-notional relations is crucial in this process. Only when coherent network of hierarchical connections is revealed, certain elements may be singled out. They can consequently be considered as potential directions for development of a particular field.

Notional model of a certain field of knowledge reveals 'a cognitive barrier', which sometimes turns out to be more difficult to overcome than 'a language barrier'. One can perfectly know a foreign language and at the same time may not be able to understand the meaning of, for instance, an article about ship building written both in his/her mother tongue and the foreign language. One may not be able to understand the meaning not because he/she does not know terms of certain lexicon but especially because the logical-notional model of a certain domain does not exist in his/her mind. Such conclusions add weight to arguments in discussion about the quality of translations done by subject-field experts and language experts, as a rule in favour of the first ones.

Nevertheless, the precise division of knowledge internalized in a human brain (mind) into language and non-language knowledge is not possible. It is just a certain simplified research assumption. Between the two distinguished phenomena some transitional forms surely exist. Taking into account the fact that such an object of research as knowledge is inaccessible to direct and thorough examination, types of knowledge mentioned above are to be considered as a certain approximation.

There is one common but incorrect belief that texts contain knowledge. In fact, as it was stated above, knowledge exists only as a certain property of living beings. The opinion that language expressions (words, statements, texts) contain knowledge is false, they do not contain knowledge but represent it (in phonetic or graphic form). Consequently, in the process of communication members of a particular speech community are able to present to other members of this community only texts (utterances). These texts represent knowledge. Understanding them according to author's intention depends on the measure of how coincident author's and receiver's idiolects are, both in the aspect of expressional and referential means – so it depends on the precision of the idiolects. A text as the form of knowledge representation is the key component of communication process, within which acts of knowledge transference are carried out. In domain-specific (professional) communication a specialist text plays this role respectively.

Discussion on the principles of human communication is present in linguistics from the very beginning. The models of communication developed in linguistics are well-known and commonly accepted (see for example F. Grucza 1983, 2009). Linguists use them as a kind of approximation that helps, among others, to develop the model of language acquisition or to find principles and techniques of translation process.

No matter what aspect of knowledge is discussed, one cannot forget about the human being, as he/she should hold the central position in deliberations both on knowledge and communication. This anthropocentric dimension of communication (and linguistics in general) is the starting point for this article and its theses.

2. Transference

Considering the problem of knowledge transference, in this article we have in mind domain-specific knowledge, including scientific knowledge, i.e. achievements of particular experts whose professional activity is focused on certain domain or field. By achievements we mean here the store of knowledge of these people, their state of mind.

Acts of knowledge transference (as well as acts of communication) are carried out through the means of certain language expressions (texts) that represent knowledge. Perceiving knowledge transference (general knowledge or scientific knowledge) as the process that is realized through production and reception (in literal meaning) of some amount of knowledge (information) is wrong. Reading the text does not mean taking the content out of the text but it means reconstructing information (knowledge) that the author wanted to express. Therefore, reconstruction means interpreting (decoding) author's intention.

Knowledge transference perceived in this way is closely related to the activity defined as reconstruction. The whole process (of transference) cannot be carried out without the means of knowledge representation, i.e. texts (specialist texts). The content of the text reconstructed (interpreted) by the receiver does not necessarily have to be (and usually is not) identical to the content (message) intended to be expressed by the sender (author). Therefore, to be understood the sender and the receiver should constantly co-ordinate the meaning of language expressions that are used by them in communication process. The sender should always have in mind the intended receiver of the text and therefore should revise knowledge according to target context. This assumes, on one hand, taking into consideration the receiver's perception ability and, on the other hand, searching for the most effective (in communication) formulas of professional knowledge.

Such an understanding of knowledge transference phenomenon has been described lately in works of Polish linguists affiliated to the Faculty of Applied Linguistics, University of Warsaw (F. Grucza 1994, 1997, 2005, 2006; B. Z. Kielar 2003; J. Lukszyn 1991, 2006). The main theses of this conception are presented below.

In the model of knowledge transference proposed by F. Grucza two main dimensions of this phenomenon are distinguished:

1. vertical transference;
2. horizontal transference.

Vertical transference is considered equivalent to knowledge popularization within one professional community in order to present achievements of some members of this community to others. In other words it means activities that make possible the 'flow' of domain-specific knowledge from more specific to less specific level. This kind of knowledge transference is done by multiplication of specialist texts of different 'expertise degree'. Taking into account the target group, texts for some reasons incomprehensible for receivers are transformed into completely comprehensible ones. Such a method supposes some simplification of knowledge represented by original texts. Consequently, so-called domain-specific translation of texts in a certain LSP is applied in this process. It can be, for instance, such a reformulation of the content that the language of the text is more comprehensible to wider audience. This kind of 'expertise degree' reduction of language means (for example in order to adapt a specialist text to teaching purposes) may result in potential knowledge deformation (see part 3. of this article).

The procedure aimed at simplification of specialist texts is core activity within popularization of scientific knowledge. The effectiveness of knowledge popularization depends on the measure how certain specialist texts could be translated into texts formulated in either simplified LSP or general language and at the same time could reflect the most important components of knowledge (concepts) represented by original texts. Such activities are firstly difficult and secondly they require great responsibility as they apply not only to expression level but also semantic level of a text. It is highly recommended to assign such work to experts with the highest competence in a certain field because they would be able to evaluate what transformations of domain-specific knowledge are acceptable (F. Grucza 1994: 46–49, 2005: 68–69).

Transference of new knowledge, i.e. its externalization by the means of a language, assumes not only transformations in the system of current knowledge but also necessity to develop ‘repository’ of expressional means, which can be so extensive that it may result in distinguishing a new LSP. It happens when new concepts appear – gathering components of knowledge within a certain field may result in changing the status of quasi-terms into terms which is reflected in one-to-one relation (each term reflects one particular notion). Linguistic accuracy (precision of terminological units in representing concepts) of the LSP is one of measures that indicate the stage of development of a certain domain (compare the history of a term *phoneme* mentioned in J. Lukszyn 1991: 85).

Horizontal transference, by contrast, refers to interdisciplinary or/and international aspect of domain-specific knowledge popularization. It aims at offering the possibility to acquaint with knowledge developed by the community of users of a certain ethnolect or LSP. This kind of transference is done through multiplication of specialist texts that are created in a certain LSP (interdisciplinary aspect) or multiplication of specialist texts that are created in a certain foreign language (international aspect).

This article refers to the second of two above-mentioned aspects of transference, i.e. international (interlingual) knowledge transference. When transference activities are carried out within speech communities and knowledge popularization gains interlingual dimension, the necessity of optimal or the most adequate translation becomes essential. In practice, it is a question that gives rise to much controversy as the problem of translation equivalence and its potential types has been discussed by linguists for a long time (B. Z. Kielar 2003). It is also worth mentioning that ‘the newer’ from receivers’ perspective is the knowledge represented by original text the more difficult is a search for equivalent translation of a specialist text. Adequate externalization of knowledge often requires development of expressional means first. This fact remains in direct relation with the question of ‘expertise degree’ of LSPs.

Interlingual perspective of knowledge transference process determines two important aspects of popularization. One of them is that transcoding knowledge through linguistic means, 'transferring' it from one language into another requires creating a corresponding LSP. Some LSPs gained the common importance and even if these are foreign languages everybody has to know them to some extent and, moreover, has to update them constantly. Another relates to popularizing knowledge that is new for a particular community. This process assumes popularization of the language that represents 'borrowed' knowledge, which may result in creating and promoting a new way of thinking among target receivers.

3. Translation

Above-mentioned aspects of knowledge transference imply two different types of barriers that hinder proper perception of specialist texts and, consequently, two types of specialist text translation. These are:

1. subject-field translation connected with cognitive barrier (unfamiliarity with the domain of knowledge);
2. interlingual translation connected with language barrier (unfamiliarity with the LSP).

Firstly, we deal with cognitive barrier and subject-field translation in the situation when the potential receiver is not able to understand the text formulated (correctly) in a certain LSP because he/she does not possess knowledge of the field. Transference of scientific knowledge in this sense is understood as adapting original texts to receivers' perceptual abilities. The fact that the receiver is not able to deal with a certain text indicates that he/she does not have enough domain-specific knowledge to reconstruct the meaning of the text. It can also result from not enough knowledge of rules of logic or intellectual traditions in a particular field. In this context arises the necessity to 'translate' texts worded in a certain LSP into texts worded in corresponding language for general purposes (LGP). So-called 'subject-field translation' from LSP into LGP affects text's 'mapping potential' (its ability to represent mental structures (concepts and relations between them) through certain language units and text's logical syntax) lowering it to some extent. The demanded degree of reduction of a certain LSP and consequent restriction of knowledge expressed through texts worded in this LSP depends on language development of a particular field of knowledge. The higher 'language specialization' of a certain domain the more serious reduction in the body of a text worded in a certain LSP is needed when popularizing knowledge of this field among wide range of receivers. It is also worth mentioning that simplification of any LSP in the process of subject-field translation results in both quantitative and qualitative 'impoverishment' of knowledge represented by original specialist texts. It can be for example lowering the level of knowledge accuracy. The more generalized specialist texts of highly developed domains become, the more ambiguous their interpretation can be. On the other hand, in the case of subject fields represented by languages that so far do not differ clearly from corresponding LGP the problem is precise differentiation between scientific texts and texts worded in a certain LGP. Consequently, within such fields of knowledge it is difficult to recognize texts that indeed present new knowledge as distinct from those that in fact popularize 'old' knowledge (F. Grucza 2002: 19–26, 2005: 69–70, 2006: 28–48).

Considering subject-field translation we can distinguish two stages of this process. The first one is creating or selecting already created language units for the piece of knowledge that is to be expressed. The second is externalization of knowledge, making it possible to be perceived by receivers. Beside language operations, the process assumes also some metalanguage operations for example defining, explication of terms etc. Therefore, subject-field translation in some aspect deals with modelling knowledge. One of the examples is encyclopaedic model that presents domain-specific (scientific) knowledge in the form of so-called secondary texts (dictionaries, encyclopaedias, lectures). Devising such a model requires certain compression of knowledge, which is eventually presented as scientific information. In consequence, any encyclopaedic model of domain-specific knowledge is derivative of many real texts and at the same time represents these texts on the basis of semantic model.

Secondly, we deal with language barrier in the situation when the potential receiver is not able to understand the text formulated in a certain LSP because he/she does not know expressional means of this LSP. Such difficulties may be solved through interlingual translation. The core question of translation is the problem of equivalence. When talking about specialist text translation it is worth mentioning that maintaining both expressional (formal) and conceptual (semantic) equivalency should be the main challenge for a translator. Nevertheless, it is highly possible that in the process of translation some transformations both in semantic and expression level of a text would occur.

As it was stated above, professional communication takes place in two different contexts, i.e. sender's context of knowledge and receiver's context of knowledge are distinguished. There are certain assumptions in reference literature concerning these two phenomena. Firstly, sender's context of knowledge and receiver's context of knowledge are not identical. They are compatible only in terms of common hypertext that is the pattern of subject-field communication. Secondly, receiver's context of knowledge is variable – it depends on the sender's context of knowledge. Thirdly, a specialist text can be thoroughly understood only in the sender's context of knowledge (J. Lukszyn 2006: 164).

Concerning semantic (conceptual) transformations that were mentioned above it is difficult to separate them from expressional means. Referents are mental units (they exist in human's mind) and it is impossible to research into them directly. Nevertheless, a mark of conceptual transformations can be traced in the text itself, through investigation of expressional means. It is assumed that in receiver's context of knowledge the content of a specialist text undergoes certain transformations. These transformations include simplification, amplification, reorganization, deformation and destruction of knowledge represented by the sender's (original) text. Three of them (simplification, amplification and reorganization of knowledge) may have both positive and negative quality. The positive effect of such knowledge transformations can be symbolically described as 'clearing up' of the text content whereas the negative effect can be referred to as 'obscuring' it. The example of negative amplification is the situation when the text is given the meaning it does not imply, for instance when a review of a scientific text is regarded as the scientific text itself. The other transformations, i.e. deformation and destruction, are negative and undesirable phenomena as their general result is impoverishment of the content of translated text (for more on this topic, see M. Małachowicz 2008).

4. Conclusions

Transference acts are the starting point of the process of knowledge popularization, the process of great importance for communication. It should be emphasized, though, that the real act of knowledge popularization is done only when the receiver understands the text according to sender's intention, in other words, when he reconstructs the meaning. Transference of new domain-specific knowledge is usually accompanied by transference of new expressional means from source language (text) to target language (text). It is due to the fact that translation of specialist texts that represent new knowledge requires certain enrichment of a target language (especially subject-field terminology).

It can be assumed, then, that knowledge popularization both in inter-domain and interlingual dimension is connected with transference of not only expressional means but also conceptual components – the elements of a certain cognitive style, i.e. the way of solving intellectual tasks. A good illustration of this phenomenon is the assumption at one time popular in cognitive sciences, which claimed that human's mind functions similarly to artificial intelligence. Research based on this assumption and its results were defined as a computer metaphor (K. Domańska 1997).

References

Domańska, K. (1997): *Metafora komupterowa w psychologii poznawczej*. In: M. Majerska/ T. Tyszka (eds), Psychologia i życie. Warszawa. 12–37.

Grucza, F. (1983): *Zagadnienia metalingwistyki*. Warszawa.

Grucza, F. (1994): *O upowszechnianiu wiedzy naukowej i jego językowych współczynnikach*. In: Nauka. 4. 31–55.

Grucza, F. (1997): *Języki ludzkie a wyrażenia językowe, wiedza a informacja, mózg a umysł ludzki*. In: F. Grucza/ M. Dakowska (eds), Podejścia kognitywne w lingwistyce, translatoryce i glottodydaktyce. Warszawa. 7–19.

Grucza, F. (2002): *Języki specjalistyczne – indykatory i/ lub determinanty rozwoju cywilizacyjnego*. In: J. Lewandowski (ed.), Problemy technolingwistyki (= Języki specjalistyczne 2). Warszawa. 9–26.

Grucza, F. (2005): *Wyrażenie „upowszechnianie nauki' – jego status i znaczenie w świetle teorii aktów komunikacyjnych i lingwistyki tekstów*. In: F. Grucza/ W. Wiśniewski (eds), Teoria i praktyka upowszechniania nauki. Warszawa. 41–74.

Grucza, F. (2006): *Glottodydaktyka: nauka – praca naukowa – wiedza*. In: Przegląd Glottodydaktyczny. 20. 5–48.

Grucza, F. (2006): *Metanaukowa i metalingwistyczna wizja lingwistyki (stosowanej)*. In: Lingwistyka Stosowana/ Applied Linguistics/ Angewandte Linguistik. 1. 19–39.

Grucza, S. (2012a): *Fachsprachenlinguistik*. Frankfurt/ M.

Grucza, S. (2012b): *Ścisłość języków specjalistycznych a ścisłość tekstów specjalistycznych*. In: K. Grzywka/ R. Małecki/ M. Filipowicz/ J. Godlewicz–Adamiec/ P. Kociumbas/ D. Wyrzykiewicz/ E. Michta (ed.), Kultura – literatura – język. Pogranicza Komparatystyki./ Kultur – Literatur – Sprache. Warszawa. 1272–1285.

Grucza, S. (2012c): *Kognitive Funktion von Fachsprachen als Gegenstand der Fachsprachenlinguistik*. In: F. Grucza/ H.-R. Spiegel/ O. Schneider-Mizony/ J. Żmudzki (eds), Akten des XII. internationalen Germanistenkongresses, Warschau 2010. Fachsprachen in Theorie und Praxis. Geschichte des Deutschen als Fremdsprachenunterricht weltweit / Geschichte von DaF weltweit. Theorie und Geschichte der Translationswissenschaft. Bd. 18. Frankfurt/ M. 31–37.

Kielar, B. Z. (2003): *Zarys translatoryki*. Warszawa.

Krzeszowski, T. P. (1997): *O znaczeniu przymiotnika „kognitywny'*. In: F. Grucza/ M. Dakowska (eds), Podejścia kognitywne w lingwistyce, translatoryce i glottodydaktyce. Warszawa. 23–31.

Lukszyn, J. (1991): *Lingwistyczne problemy badań terminologicznych*. In: F. Grucza (ed.), Teoretyczne podstawy terminologii. Wrocław. 79–95.

Lukszyn, J. (2006): *Zasady analizy tekstów specjalistycznych*. In: A. Wołodźko–Butkiewicz/ W. Zmarzer (eds), Glottodydaktyka i jej konteksty interkulturowe. Warszawa. 161–171.

Małachowicz, M. (2008): *Transfer wiedzy specjalistycznej w układzie interlingwalnej komunikacji zawodowej*. University of Warsaw. Warszawa (unpublished PhD Thesis).

NEP (2004): *Nowa encyklopedia powszechna PWN*. Warszawa.

STP (2005): J. Lukszyn (ed.), *Języki specjalistyczne. Słownik terminologii przedmiotowej*. Warszawa.

Could Eye-Tracking Help to Reconstruct the Translation Processes?

Ewa Zwierzchoń-Grabowska (University of Warsaw)

1. Emergence of eye-tracking-based translation research

In recent years several research centres in Poland which deal with issues of translation have launched a new type of instrumental translation studies, that is translation studies employing a video-based eye-tracking device. The emergence of such studies results from development of a technology that enables observation of certain translation-oriented aspects.

Eye-tracking-oriented translation studies are currently conducted at the Faculty of Applied Linguistics of Warsaw University, namely at the Institute of Culturology and Anthropocentric Linguistics, in the Laboratory of Experimental Eye-tracking Linguistics (LELO), in the Applied Linguistics Institute at the Audiovisual Translation Laboratory (AVT Lab), at the Catholic University of Lublin in the Psycho-Neuro-Physiological Laboratory and the Studio High Definition, at the Adam Mickiewicz University of Poznań and the UMCS of Lublin. In these centres, research concerning audiovisual translation, audio description, sight translation and written translation is conducted (see S. Grucza 2011, 2012a, 2012b, 2012c; I. Mazur/A. Chmiel 2011; I. Krejtz et al. 2012a, 2012b, M. Płużyczka 2011a, 2011b, 2012a, 2012b, 2012c; E. Zwierzchoń 2011).

(1) Interlingual translations: sight translation and written translation

In interlingual translation a text made in one language (source text) is translated into a text made in another language (target language). The communication situation with the presence of a translator is shown in the diagram of the translational system:

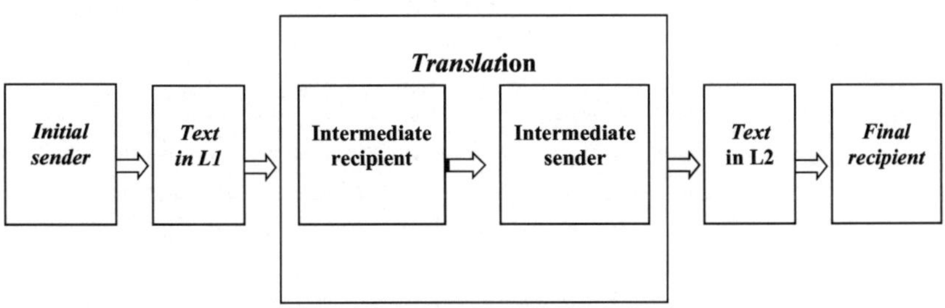

Diagram 1: Translation system (cf. F. Grucza 1981)

This model pertains both to the situation in which text in L1 has written or spoken form and a situation in which text in L2 has written or spoken form. Depending on the modal form of the text, four variants of interlingual translations may be specified, but only two of them: sight translation and written translation are currently analysed using eye-tracking techniques. In sight translation, the source text (text in L1) has written form, and the target text (text in L2) has spoken form. When both the source text (text in L1) and the target text (text in L2) have written form, we encounter a typical written translation.

It is also possible to encounter a translation set in which the source text (text in L1) has spoken form, and the target text (text in L2) has written form. It is the rarest of all situations as the source text in spoken form to be translated into the target text in written form is usually written down beforehand, and it is rendered for translation in written form. This type of translation is not currently subject to eye-tracking analysis, even though it would be possible taking into account the presence of the visual factor. When both the source text (text in L1) and the target text (text in L2) have spoken form, we encounter interpreting. But interpreting is not subject to eye-tracking tests taking into account the lack of a visual factor.

(2) Interlingual audiovisual translation

In audiolingual translation the source text may as well have the form of written or spoken text and the source text may as well have the form of written or spoken text. In addition to that, there is an image which the translator must take into account when translating. Among types of audiovisual translation one may enumerate also audio description (AD) and developing subtitles for the deaf and hard-of-hearing (SDH) as well as intersemiotic audiovisual translations (see T. Tomaszkiewicz 2010).

(3) Audio description

Audio description is intended for final recipients who are not able to see the visual elements of film. Yet one should point out that in the case of audio description instead of a text (linguistic signs), the object of translation ('description') is an image (non-linguistic visual signs), and the target text has spoken form (linguistic audial signs).

The text that results from audio description may still be a source text to be further translated by the translator. From a general perspective a text made in L1 in spoken form (source text) is translated into a text made in L2 also in spoken form. In translation practice a translator may be required to translate a text both in spoken or written form. Similarly, a text in L2 made by the translator may have spoken or written form. That is why depending on the form of the source text and the form of the target text made by the translator translating audio description may be interlingual audiovisual translation – oral and oral, oral and written, written and written, written and oral.

(4) Subtitles for the deaf and hard of hearing

A similar situation pertains to subtitles for the deaf and hard of hearing. Linguistic audial signs made in L1 may be subject to 'translation' into linguistic visual signs (subtitles) made in the same L1. It is then intralingual translation. Non-linguistic audial signs (various sounds) may be subject to 'translation' into visual linguistic signs (subtitles) made in L1. Thus, it is intersemiotic translation. In both cases the target text has written form.

Similarly in that case the developed subtitles for the deaf and hard of hearing may be a source text to be translated by the translator. In translation practice, the source text to be translated by the translator also has written form and the target text developed by the translator has written form. Thus, it is written interlingual translation; and considering that the translator must take into account also the image, it is audiovisual written interlingual translation.

2. The subject of eye-tracking test

The prerequisite for an eye-tracking test using a eye-tracker is the presence of a visual factor whose perception may be tested using the eye-tracker. This may be an image or source text or target text in written form. Following the above presentation, not all types of translation meet that condition. Typical (non-audiovisual) interlingual interpreting (that is oral and oral) does not meet that condition and this is why it is not subject to testing using a (video)eye-tracker. An eye-tracker may be used to test sight translation, written translation, audiovisual translation, audio description and subtitles for the deaf.

Nevertheless, one should point out that in the tests analysing sight translation or written translation the subject tested using the eye-tracker is the translator, that is, the movements of their eyeballs. Testing the final recipient should not be ruled out, but one may observe that it is the translator who is tested in the ongoing studies analysing the process.

Still, in eye-tracking tests analysing audiovisual interlingual translation, audio description or subtitling for the deaf and hard of hearing it is the final recipient who is subject to the test. Next, on the grounds of gained data concerning the eyeball movements of the final recipient, conclusions concerning activities of another person – the translator in audiovisual interlingual translation, audio descriptor or descriptor developing subtitles for the deaf – are drawn.

Also in this case, testing the translator in the process of audiovisual interlingual translation, the audio descriptor or descriptor developing subtitles for the deaf and hard of hearing using an eye-tracker cannot be ruled out. Nevertheless, one may note that in the ongoing studies concerning that process it is the final recipient who is analysed, and not the translator.

3. Eyeball movements

Eye-tracking analysis makes it possible to monitor the movements of the subject's eyeballs as well as points (spots) that the subject is gazing at. The prerequisite for eye-tracking tests is, as mentioned before, the presence of a visual element. This is why that eye-tracking may be used to analyse sight translation, written translation, audiovisual translation, audio description, that is types of translation containing a visual element.

One should point out that not all eyeball movements are subject to monitoring in eye-tracking translation studies. Generally, in eye-tracking research one differentiates many types of eyeball movements, such as saccades, microsaccades, smooth pursuits, nystagmus, non-movement phases (minimal movements), so called fixations. Moreover, one differentiates horizontal, vertical and torsional movements, convergent and divergent movements, conscious and subconscious movements etc.

Depending on the aim of the study, various parameters of the movements are recorded and analysed. Eye-tracking translation studies focus on the observation of fixations and saccades, and in the case of motion images – additionally on smooth pursuits. What is essential for these studies is not so much eyeball movements and their types, but non-movement moments of eyeballs (minimal movements), that is fixations, and to be more precise the spots on which the subject's eyes concentrated during a fixation. Another important type of movement in translation studies is shifting eyesight from the spot of fixation to the spot in which another fixation takes place. Also important are refixations, that is repeated fixations on the same spot and regressions, that is regressive saccades. Monitoring these types of movement results from the aim of the studies and theoretical assumptions. The most frequently analysed parameters of the movements include the duration of fixations, their position, frequency, repeated fixations on the same spots, duration of saccades, their distance, direction, frequency of repetition. Eye-tracking makes it possible to record and measure all these parameters. An important advantage of eye-tracker-based tests is their non-contact nature. Another advantage is ease of use, both for the tester and the subject tested. Owing to that fact, a higher number of research subjects may be obtained and the tests are becoming more widely spread. What is more, the test may be conducted anywhere, not only in specialist laboratories, obviously on condition that relevant rules are observed to guarantee the accuracy of the test so that the test could really measure what is to be tested.

Testing solely eyeball movements of an interpreter in the process of interpreting, that is without a visual element on which their gaze would be fixed, is also possible, but it requires that the study be based on other theoretical assumptions than in the case of the studies described above. One should also consider application of another eye-tracking method than video-based eye-tracking, e.g. electrooculography that makes it possible to monitor the eyeball movements with eyes closed.

4. The potential of eye tracker-based research of translation

The above examples show that translation studies using the eye-tracking methodology are varied. Later on we will focus on one type of translation specified above, namely on non-audiovisual written interlingual translation, that is translation of a written text in L1 into a text in L2 that also has written form. It is worth adding that in that case only the text as such is subject to translation without any images, clips or sounds.

At the very beginning one should underline that the proper object of the studies described is the process of translation that occurs in the brain of the translator while translating a text in L1 into a text in L2. The process is not available for direct observation, and conclusions concerning its course are drawn using the observable factors that are connected with it. The framework of the studies discussed in this part is limited to the observation of the eyeballs of the translator at the moment of translation. In the presented case both text in L1 and text in L2 have written form, thus a visual factor is present. Additionally, both texts are in written form displayed on the screen of an eye-tracker, and the translator translates using specific computer software. It is then a typical written translation, that is translating a written text into a written text (see B.Z. Kielar 2003: 129), and the fact that the translator uses texts in electronic form and translates them using a computer are important assumptions because they are the prerequisite for testing that uses an eye-tracker of a given type – a eye tracker.

With reference to the translation system one may point out that eye-tracking studies make it possible to record the movements of eyeballs of the initial sender, translator or final recipient. The initial sender may be subject to such monitoring while they produce text in L1, and the translator - when they receive text in L1, while they translate and while they produce text in L2; the final recipient may be monitored while they receive text in L2.

In that case, however, the range of eye-tracking translation studies is limited to monitoring the translator, that is the stage of text in L1 reception by the translator, the translation stage and the stage of text in L2 development by the translator. We eliminate though the first and last of the above-mentioned stages, that is monitoring the initial sender and monitoring the final recipient.

The stage of development by the initial sender of text in L1 is basically a process of text writing and it should be analysed as such a process. It takes place in the brain of the initial sender, i.e. person other than the translator, and it depends on the properties of that person and not of the translator. Similarly, the text B reception stage by the final recipient, that is also a person other than the translator, is a process of text reading and depends on the properties of that person and not the translator. These processes were researched among others by M.A. Just/P. A. Carpenter (1980), I. Kurcz/A. Polkowska (1990), K. Rayner (1998).

As results from the above, the study in question pertains only to a part of the translational system, which may be illustrated by the following figure:

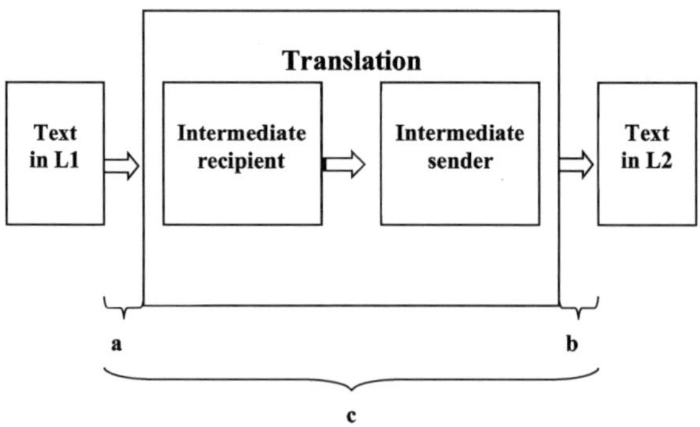

Diagram 2: Own compilation using the work of F. Grucza (1981)

- Text in L1 is an input text in written form in L1 displayed on the screen of a eye–tracker;
- Text in L2 is a target text recorded by the translator in written form in L2 and displayed on the screen of a eye–tracker;
- a – recording the movements of the translator's eyeballs when their gaze is directed to the area of text in L1;
- b – recording the movements of the translator's eyeballs when their gaze is directed to the area of text in L2;
- c – recording the movements of the translator's eyeballs when their gaze is being shifted from the area of text in L1 to the area of text in L2.

Tests using the eye-tracker are non-invasive tests. They employ a camera integrated with the monitor of an eye-tracker that records the infrared light motion reflected by the eye. The subject translates text in L1 into text in L2 using a computer like in a real-life situation, and simultaneously the eye-tracker records the movements of the subject's eyeballs.

The difference between a real-life situation in which the translator renders a text and the test situation is that during the test dedicated eye-tracker software runs at the same time as the software which the subject uses and that the monitor is not a regular computer monitor but it is equipped with a special camera. The operation of the additional software is invisible for the subject and has no influence on the translation in progress. The presence of the camera may be noticed to the extent that the test is preceded by a calibration procedure and it requires keeping a given distance from the eye-tracker screen. Moreover, the subjects are informed about the academic aim of the test and their participation is voluntary. Taking into account a limited number of eye-trackers, the test is usually carried out in a dedicated room. The subjects are then aware that they participate in a test, but the external conditions are very similar to a real-life situation. Translating a written text made accessible to the translator in electronic form into a written text also in electronic form is currently a typical translation practice. The test is then conducted in conditions that resemble a real-life situation, which decreases the risk that the obtained test-based data will significantly differ from real parameters. Using a different type of eye-tracker for testing the process of written translation, for instance a mobile eye-tracker, electrooculograph or special attachments to the eye would require placing some kind of device on the subject's head, attaching electrodes, or placing a special lens on the eyeball, which would lead to a significant change in external conditions in which a translator works.

Studies whose object is the process of translation are difficult to conduct in that respect that the researcher may not observe the very object of research directly. The researcher draws conclusions concerning the process on the basis of their knowledge of the input text, external factors (conditions) that influence the translation process and the translated text that is the result of the translation process as well as its perception by the final recipient.

Eye-tracking tests conducted using a state-of-the-art apparatus like a eye-tracker will surely not guarantee a complete cognition of the written translation process, but they will help to obtain data that will contribute to a better knowledge of the process. The very translation process that occurs in the brain of the translator remains unavailable for direct observation by the researcher.

What may be observed, or to be more precise recorded, by the eye-tracker is only the movement of the translator's eyeballs while translating a written text or of the eyeballs of the recipient of the translated text. Nevertheless, data obtained through the tests using a eye-tracker may expand the knowledge of researchers with previously unknown information and allow them notice the phenomena which will either help to verify the current theories or develop a new theory or, at the functional level, develop effective tools to assist the translator in the translation process or to optimize the process of educating written translators.

4.1. Research questions regarding the process of translation

Using the eye tracker device makes it possible to conduct a quantitative examination and to undertake a statistical analysis which would suffice to provide answers to the following essential research questions:

- How do the translator's eyeballs move during the translation of written text in L1 into written text in L2?
- Due to the complexity of the process studied it seems necessary to pose, along with the main question above, also the following additional research questions:
- How do the translator's eyeballs move during the translation of written text into another written text when receiving text in L1?
- How do the translator's eyeballs move during the translation of written text into another written text when writing text in L2?
- How do the translator's eyeballs move during the translation of a written text into another written text when moving their eyes from text in L1 to text in L2?
- Is the eyeball movement of the translator rendering a written text into another written text when receiving text in L1 different from the eyeball movement when producing text in L2? Or how does the eyeball movement of the translator rendering a written text into another written text when receiving text in L1 differ from the eyeball movement when producing text in L2?
- Can characteristic fixation sequences be observed?
- Can any regular patterns of fixation on specific elements of text bc observed, e.g. conjunctions, pronouns, abbreviations, numbers, etc.?
- How long are the phrases translated ‘at one time’ and what does their length depend on?
- How often and in which cases does the translator move their eyes to a part of the text further than the currently translated fragment?
- How often does the subject move their eyes from text in L1 to text in L2?
- How long does moving the eyes from text in L1 to text in L2 take and vice versa?
- What is the translation speed? Does it change, and if so, how does it change during the translation?

4.2. Optimization of translator's tools

In the eye-tracking tests in which the translator renders the text with the use of computer software it is also necessary to consider the particular software. The history of machine translation, including the development of various computer programmes used in translation, was presented by J. Hutchings (1995). An area which merits particular attention is the research into translation memories and currently developed Computer Aided Translation (CAT) tools, such as Trados – by TRADOS GmbH, a company founded in 1984, which began its work on the translation support software already in 1980's, was subsequently taken over by the British company SDL and which developed SDL Trados Studio 2009; Wordfast – developed in 1999, with its currently most popular version Wordfast Classic, since 2009 also offered as Wordfast Translation Studio; OmegaT – developed in 2000 in C++, and in 2001 in the Java language; DejaVu of 1993, or MemoQ by Kilgray, a company established in 2004. Trados (SDL Trados Studio 2009), Wordfast (Wordfast Translation Studio), OmegaT, DejaVu, MemoQ are currently the most popular CAT tools.

On the other hand, the eye-tracking research must undoubtedly exclude those programmes which automatically translate written texts, i.e. on the basis of a text in L1 generate a text in L2 without any human input, the so called ‘automated translators’. In the use of such programmes the translator's contribution is only limited to specifying the text which is to be translated and the language into which the translation is to be made. The translator does not render the text, thus it is impossible to conduct the eye-tracking research of the process. It is the following translational system:

Text in L1 → computer software → Text in L2

The CAT software mentioned above, which is intended to assist written translators, may, however, be used in the eye-tracking research. There may be identified two basic variants of translating text in L1 into text in L2 with the use of CAT tools. In the first variant, during the rendition of the text the translator uses various tools available in the computer software to facilitate text translation.

Text in L1 → translator + computer software → Text in L2

In the other variant, the computer software generates a preliminary version of the translation, which is then improved, supplemented or corrected by the translator.

Text in L1 → computer software → preliminary Text in L2 → translator → Text in L2

Moreover, with the use of CAT tools, the translation may be performed by the translator individually or in collaboration with other translators within a local network or over the Internet. In both these variants the translator translates a written electronic text into another written electronic text, therefore an eye-tracking research of such process is possible. However, the fact that in each of those variants the translation process is carried out differently must be taken into account and, thus, each of them must be studied individually. Only at the next stage is it possible to compare the results of each individual study, which would allow for the formulation of conclusions as to the whether, depending on the CAT tool used, the performance of the translation process is or is not optimal.

The second type of software, which may be used in eye-tracking research, are text processors, such as the popular Writer or Microsoft Word, that is non-translation software, which translators yet often use in translating written texts. The basic function of such programmes is text editing, however, they are also equipped with functions useful in the act of translation, such as opening two texts at the same time in two separate windows, one above the other or side by side, simultaneous scrolling of two texts, searching, replacing, recording macros, etc.

Due to the use of computer software during the translation, also with respect to this scope of the process studied, the following research questions may be posed:

- Are the places of fixation, sequences of fixations and saccades, the scanpath from text in L1 to text in L2 and from text in L2 to text in L1, the translation time or other parameters measurable in an eye-tracking research different or the same in the case the translator uses different software? If differences occur, what causes them?
- Can the translation process employed by translators in the case of written translations involving computer software be improved and, if so, how? That is, how to develop computer software in order to most effectively support the translator in the process of translating written texts?

The aim of the eye-tracking research into the written translation process of a translator who uses computer translation software may also be to compare and evaluate various computer translation software or to develop criteria to evaluate the CAT tools with respect to their optimality for the translator's eye movement. In the existing comparisons of computer translation software only the functionalities of such software are compiled, i.e. information on whether a particular functionality is or is not featured in the given software. Sometimes user opinions on the functionality are mentioned – whether it is useful, convenient, quick to find, and so on. Such user opinions are a source of certain feedback to the authors of such software, however, they are only subjective and imprecise valuations, mostly basing on intuition and not comparable criteria. The eye-tracking research could provide objective data, gained in the course of a systematic research, which would facilitate the development of translation software supporting the written translator in their translation process in the most effective manner.

Apart from the computer software listed above, which may be used by the translator during the act of translation, one other type of computer software merits attention, namely the translodidactic programmes or platforms which are used in translation didactics, as for instance the intelligent Web-based didactic models for translation training developed as part of the LISTiG project (see S. Grucza 2010). Their main purpose is to be used in an effective translation learning process, and not during translation itself, yet the main parameters measured in the course of the process, such as the place and duration of fixation, regressions, sequences of fixations and saccades, the duration of saccades, etc. apply to both the written translation rendered by a professional translator with appropriately high translation competence level, as well as to the translation rendered during exercises intending to develop the translation competence.

Moreover, it must be noted that during the translation process the translator has access to the entire text in language A, however, depending on the length of the text, can see either the whole or a part of the text only. In the case of a text in an electronic form, which is translated on the computer, the length of the visible text depends on whether the entire text or only a part of it may be displayed on the monitor. Usually the length of the translated text and the technical specifications of the monitor: its screen size, resolution and graphic capabilities of the software, allow for only a part of the text to be displayed. Analogous possibilities and constraints apply to the length of the visible target text in language B, with the exception that during the translation process the translator may only see that part of the target text they have already translated and typed. The entire target text may only be visible after it has been typed by the translator and only if it fits onto the screen, otherwise merely a part of such text is visible (displayed).

The size and location of the visible parts of text in L1 and text in L2 with respect to each other is of key importance to eye-tracking research, as only the visible parts of texts in L1 and L2 are examined. At the same time the size and location of the visible parts of text in L1 and text in L2 with respect to each other may be an important factor during text translation. With regard to the size of the field of texts in L1 and L2 the following research questions may be formulated:

- What is the optimal length of the displayed part of the source text, that is how long a fragment of the source text should be visible to the translator during the translation process? What is the minimum length of the displayed fragment of the source text?

- What is the optimal length of the displayed part of the target text, that is how long a fragment of the target text should be visible to the translator during the translation process? What is the minimum length of the displayed fragment of the target text?

Further, the selected research materials and analysis of the translator's eye-ball movement when shifting their gaze from text in L1 to text in L2 may enable researchers to ascertain:

- The optimal spatial pattern of a text field in L1 with respect to a text field in L2, i.e. text field in L1 above text field in L2, text field in L1 below text field in L2, text field in L1 to the left of text field in L2, text field in L1 to the right of text field in L2, alternating text fields in L1 and text fields in L2, where text field in L1 is located before a corresponding text field in L2, alternating text fields in L1 and text fields in L2, where text field in L1 follows the corresponding text field in L2?

The possible locations are illustrated in the following diagram:

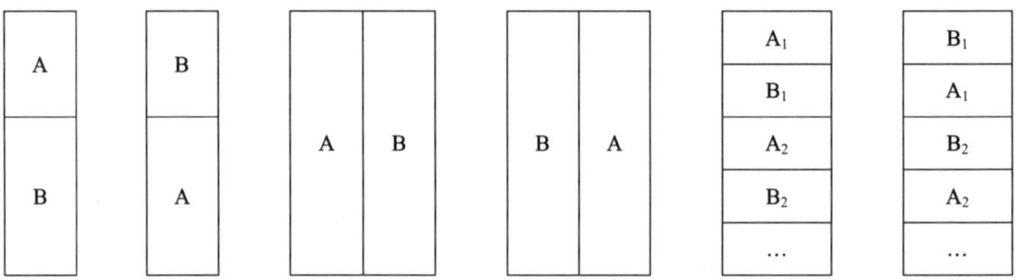

Diagram 3. Own compilation

By recording the eyeball movement the eye-tracking research provides information on the places on which the translator's eyes fixate, the duration of such fixation, the the paths along which the translator's gaze shifted, re-fixations and repetitive fixation sequences, etc. It must, however, be noted that by recording the translator's eyeball movement the eye-tracking research, on the one hand, marks the places of fixation, records the fixation sequences or the path along which the translator's eyes scanned text in L1, and on the other hand marks the places of fixation, records the fixation sequences or the path along which the translator's eyes scanned text in L2. On top of that, it records the path along which the translator's eyes shifted from text in L1 to text in L2, the places of fixation at the time, if any, fixation sequences, etc.

4.3. Supplementing research into the written translation process with other eye-tracking research

In the case of combining the eye-tracking research into the written translation process with research into other processes, such as sight translation or reading, even more complex research questions may be formulated:

- Does the reception (perception) of source text by the translator producing a written translation (of written text in L1 into written text in L2) differ – in terms of eyeball movement – from the reception (perception) of source text by the translator performing a sight translation (written text in L1 into orally produced text in L2) and if so, how?
- Does the process of reading text in L1 by the translator, who was given a particular text to translate, differ – in terms of eyeball movement – from the process of reading text in L1 by a reader, whose aim is to become acquainted with its contents and if so, how?
- Does the process of reading text in L2 by the translator who has written the particular text differ – in terms of eyeball movement – from the process of reading the same text by another person with the purpose of becoming acquainted with its contents and if so, how?

4.4. Supplementing eye-tracking research with other instrumental studies

The written translation process is a complex one, and, as the reflections presented above prove, many research questions as to its course and determining factors may be posed, which have yet remained unanswered. This article formulates over a dozen essential research questions, which will probably be answered after the relevant eye-tracking research has been concluded and its results analysed. At the same time, it must be emphasised that, owing to technological progress new instrumental translation research possibilities arise, which is, undoubtedly, a challenge for the researchers in this field.

In the future it would be interesting to combine the eye-tracking research with the research into brain activity, i.e. simultaneous observation of translator's eyeball movement and brain activity during translation.

To a certain degree the contemporary neuroimaging techniques, such as electroencephalography, or EEG, magnetoencephalography (MEG), positron emission tomography (PET), functional magnetic resonance imaging (fMRI), already make it possible to observe brain activity and provide comprehensive information with respect to the processes within the brain, i.e. the place of the activity, its intensity, but such data is yet insufficient to fully discover the language or translation processes carried out in the brain.

Nevertheless, the combination of eye-tracking research and neuroimaging could perhaps provide answers to such questions as:

- What is the brain activity during fixation?
- Is the brain activity during re-fixation the same or different?
- In the case of a repeated fixation sequence, is the brain activity the same or different? Etc.

More advanced research could help to verify the hypothesis fundamental for the eye-tracking research, and also for the research into the written translation process described here, i.e. *The Eye-Mind Hypothesis* by Marcel A. Just and Patricia A. Carpenter (see I. Kurcz/A. Polkowska 1990). Nevertheless, such research, even if possible in the future, vastly exceeds the scope of research addressed in this article.

5. Results

Tests with the use of a video-based eye-tracking device provides such data regarding the translator's eyeball movement as: (a) fixations: fixation number, duration, place, compilation of total fixation time, scanpaths, (b) regressions: number of regressions, places of re-fixations, duration of re-fixations, (c) saccades: number of saccades, duration of saccades, distance between saccades, compilation of total saccade time.

The basic methods of rendering the above results are: (i) heat maps showing the number of fixations or their duration, while the more fixations on a given place or the longer their duration, the darker (warmer) the colour of marking; (ii) gaze opacity maps, that is the more fixations on a given place or the longer their duration, the more transparent the place; (iii) focus maps highlighting the areas where the gaze falls, while the remaining areas are darkened; (iv) gaze plots, that is graphical representations showing the order and duration of fixation; (v) statistics, tables, diagrams. It is also possible to define the so called areas of interest, that is specified regions, as well as to record the data and present the results for those specified regions only.

The advantage of eye-tracking research is that it is able to objectively record the eyeball movement in all subjects. The resulting data may be statistically analysed and provide the statistical mean values of the parameters measured, scatter of results, modal value, median, standard deviation, etc. However, neither the eye tracker, nor the statistical analysis of the data gathered using it, can explain the examined phenomenon.

Only having compiled this data, which must be suitably accurate, can a researcher make inferences of the cognitive processes occurring in the translator's brain during written translation. In order to ensure the accuracy of research, it is advisable to carry out a check analysis of the data gained to ascertain whether the recorded data, e.g. place of fixation, regressions, scanpaths, gaze shifts during saccades is motivated by translation, or whether the researcher can state with absolute certainty that it has no connection with the translation and including it indiscriminately in the analysis may negatively affect the research accuracy.

The qualitative analysis of the data gained, its classification, or making inferences of the cognitive processing of translation is not unequivocal and not necessarily objective. The places of fixation occurring in all subjects or in the decided majority of subjects point to a certain regularity, yet it is the researcher's task to explain it. Explaining why a given regularity does not appear in all subjects or why some places of fixation decidedly differ in various subjects seems to be an even more complex task. Similar difficulties apply to the qualitative analysis of other parameters measured with the use of the eye tracker, i.e. duration of fixation, the path along which the translator's gaze shifted, re-fixations, repeated fixation sequences, etc. For instance, a recorded fixation, that is the subject holding the gaze on a certain element of text in L1, may be conditioned by translation, but may also be caused by a factor not related to or only indirectly related to the translation process, e.g. a recalled memory, problems with reading a word or a part of a word, glare on the monitor, momentary loss of concentration, or any other physical discomfort to the translator. Moreover, while all subjects are translators or future translators (depending on the study group), they are different in many respects, have different level of L1 competence, different knowledge of facts stated in text in L1, different level of L2 competence, different level of translation competence, etc.

Properly conducted study should be independent of any external factors, but in practice it is virtually impossible to exclude them, therefore it is important to identify such factors and either ignore certain results determined by them or properly account for them in the analysis. Eye-tracking research is often complemented by other research methods, such as questionnaire-based surveys, thinking aloud, retrospection, dialog protocols. The triangulation of methods facilitates proper interpretation of the gathered data, however, it must be remembered that, as far as eye-tracking research (recording the eyeball movement) is objective, the questionnaire-based survey, thinking aloud, retrospection, dialog protocols may be prone to error resulting from the subjective perspective of the tested person. Only after a preliminary check analysis of the data has been completed can the data be described and subsequently interpreted, and can the detailed questions be answered, such as:

- Why did the fixations occur exactly at these particular places in thc text, on these particular units? What differentiates those units, what links them?
- On what does the fixation duration depend?
- Is there a relation between the place of fixation or regressions and the lack of lexical knowledge?
- What causes regressions? Does the translator return to those places which have already been translated? How often do they do that? What causes it?
- What factors influence the speed of translation?
- How can the translator's rendition of a text be accelerated?

The above questions require the researcher's interpretation of the collected data to be answered and may also be prone to error resulting from the researcher's subjective assessment.

6. Conclusions

To conclude the above reflections it may be said that eye tracking may help in the reconstruction of written translation processes. Owing to the application of eye-tracking methodology in translation studies data may be obtained, gathering of which would not be possible with translational research methods used to date. These are, admittedly, not the parameters which directly relate to the course of the translation process occurring in the translator's brain. They concern the externally discernible behaviour of the translator during the rendition on a text, but discernible only in instrumental research, in this case the video-based eyetracking. Until now conclusions referring to the course of written translation have only been formulated basing on the analysis of the products of translator's work or their perception by a final recipient, while in the eye-tracking research the researcher's attention focuses on the person of the translator. The eye-tracking research may expand knowledge of scientists who research written translation processes with previously unknown information and enable them to observe phenomena which might allow them to verify previous theories, produce a new theory or, at the functional level, develop effective tools to assist the translator in the translation process, or optimise the process of educating written translators.

References

Just, M. A./ P. A. Carpenter (1980): *A theory of reading: From eye fixations to comprehension.* In: Psychological Review. 87. 329–354.

Grucza, F. (1980): *Zagadnienia translatoryki.* In: F. Grucza (ed.) Glottodydaktyka a translatoryka. Warszawa. 9–29.

Grucza, S. (2010): *Nowe narzędzia dydaktyki translacji: Lingwistycznie Inteligentne Systemy Translo– i Glottodydaktyczne (LISTiG).* In: Lingwistyka Stosowana/ Applied Linguistics/ Angewandte Linguistik. 3. 167–176.

Grucza, S. (2011): *Lingwistyka antropocentryczna a badania okulograficzne.* In: Lingwistyka Stosowana/ Applied Linguistics/ Angewandte Linguistik. 4. 149–162.

Grucza, S. (2012a): *The Investigation of Translation Competences and Translation Processes*, (w:) Vestnik MGLU (in press).

Grucza, S. (2012b): *Grundzüge der Anthropozentrischen Translatorik.* In: Linguistica Silesiana. An international journal of linguistic studies. (in press).

Grucza, S. (2012c): *Heat maps, gaze plots . . . and what next? The access to translation competences and translation processes.* In: S. Grucza/ M. Płużyczka/ J. Zając (eds), Translation Studies and Eye-Tracking Analysis. Frankfurt/ M. (in press).

Grucza, S./ M. Płużyczka/ J. Zając (2012): *Eye-Tracking Supported Translation Studies at the University of Warsaw (Instead of Introduction).* In: S. Grucza/ M. Płużyczka/ J. Zając (eds), Translation Studies and Eye–Tracking Analysis. Frankfurt/ M. (in press).

Hutchins, W. J. (1995): *Tłumaczenie maszynowe. Krótka historia*, [fragment książki tłumaczony na j. polski przez Annę Sosnowską]. In: E. F. K. Koerner/ R. E. Asher (eds), Concise history of the language science: from the Sumerians to the cognitivists. Oxford. 431–445. [www.mlingua.pl, 25.07.2011].

Kielra, B. Z. (2003): *Zarys translatoryki.* Warszawa.

Kurcz, I./ A. Polkowska (1990): *Interakcyjne i autonomiczne przetwarzanie informacji językowych. Na przykładzie procesu rozumienia tekstu czytanego na głos.* Wrocław.

Kreiz, I./ A. Szarkowska/ K. Kreiz/ A. Walczak/ A. Duchowski (2012a): *Audio description as an aural guide of children's visual attention: evidence form an eye-tracking study.* In: ETRA '12 Proceedings of the Symposium on Eye Tracking Research and Applications, ACM. New York, NY. 99–106. [http://dl.acm.org/citation.cfm?doid=2168556.2168572 23.10.2012].

Kreitz, K./ A. Szarkowska/ I. Kreitz/ A. Duchowski/ A. Walczak (2012b): *Multimodal learning with audio description: an eye tracking study of children's gaze during a visual recognition task.* In: Proceedings of the ACM Symposium on Applied Perception (SAP '12). ACM. New York, NY. 83–90. [http://doi.acm.org/10.1145/ 2338676.2338694 23.10.2012]

Mazur, I./ A. Chmiel (2011): *Odzwierciedlenie percepcji osób widzących w opisie dla osób niewidomych. Badania okulograficzne nad audiodeskrypcją.* In: Lingwistyka Stosowana/ Applied Linguistics/ Angewandte Linguistik. 4. 163–180.

Płużyczka, M. (2011a): *Okulograficzne wsparcie badań nad procesem tłumaczenia a'vista*, (w:) Lingwistyka Stosowana/ Applied Linguistics/ Angewandte Linguistik. 4. 181–190.

Płużyczka, M. (2011b), *Eye-Tracking Analysen in der Translationswissenschaft. Zum Stand der Forschung*, (w:) Kwartalnik Neofilologiczny. LVIII. 4/ 2011. 473–484.

Płużyczka, M. (2012a): *Na co patrzy, a co widzi tłumacz a vista? Translatoryczne możliwości poznawcze okulografii.* In: Lingwistyka Stosowana/ Applied Linguistics/ Angewandte Linguistik. 5. 66–77.

Płużyczka, M. (2012b): *Eye-tracking Support of Translation Processes Analysis.* In: Vestnik MGLU (in prcss).

Płużyczka, M. (2012c): *Eye-tracking supported research into sight translation. Lapsological conclusions.* In: S. Grucza/ M. Płużyczka/ J. Zając (eds), Translation Studies and Eye-Tracking Analysis. Frankfurt/ M. (in press).

Rayner, K. (1998). *Eye movements in reading and information processing: 20 years of research.* In: Psychological Bulletin. 124. 372–422.

Tomaszkiewicz, T. (2010): *Przekład audiowizualny, werbo–wizualny czy intersemiotyczny: różne wymiary tej samej rzeczywistości?* In: Lingwistyka Stosowana/ Applied Linguistics/ Angewandte Linguistik. 3. 33–44.

Zwierzchoń–Grabowska, E. (2011), *Okulograficzne wsparcie badań nad procesem tłumaczenia pisemnego.* In: Lingwistyka Stosowana/ Applied Linguistics/ Angewandte Linguistik. 4. 199–210.

Eye-Tracking Methods and Measures

Paweł Soluch (Neuro Devise, Warsaw)
Adam Tarnowski (University of Warsaw)

When over a hundred years ago visual attention first aroused interest its study was aided by any possible techniques available at the time. It was eye observation or introspection, which are less than precise methods for recording such partially automatic processes as eye movement.

To carry out observations during reading a system of mirrors was used, magnifying glasses, or even a telescope. An extreme example of such methods is attaching reflecting elements to the eyes and recording the light deflections on a photosensitive tape (N. Wade/B.W. Tatler 2005). The studies – perhaps owing to their limitations described above – concentrated on the movements as such, and not on the fixations. The measurement techniques developed in the direction of recording all types of eye movement. Due to the limited space of one chapter we shall only briefly present the eye-tracking study methodology, techniques and the scope of the context in which eye-tracking devices are currently employed.

When beginning your adventure with eye-tracking, you must learn several important rules governing the human visual system – the features which must always be taken into account when preparing an experiment or getting down to analyse the eye-tracking study results. These rules hold the key to understanding what eye-tracking really is. In this part we would like to concentrate on the very nature of eye movement study and description of the visual system. We believe that eye-tracking as a method can be of interest to researchers for a handful of reasons. First of all, the eye movement is probably the commonest potentially intentional human behaviour – it occurs three times per second on average. Secondly, it precisely indicates what information is being received by the subject at the given time. Thirdly, at last, control of the eye movement unquestionably constitutes a model example of cooperation between automatic and controlled mechanisms, both in the aspect of perception as well as action.

A human being can precisely observe a mere 1.5 degrees of the visual field. This roughly corresponds to the width of a word in the read text. Differentiating several visual fields (foveal visual field, parafoveal visual field and peripheral visual field) is very useful, as each of them is responsible for the reception of different visual information (S. P. Liversedge/J. M. Findlay 2000). A foveal visual field and parafoveal visual field are in charge of gathering precise information on the surroundings and identifying objects. A peripheral visual field is linked to perception and evaluation of new objects, orientation in space and the balance system. This division also results from the differences in the structure of the retina, the involvement of heterogeneous brain structures in processing concrete information provided by these fields, as well as the existence of different control mechanisms.

To clearly see the space in front of us, the visual system uses the attentional processes. Acting as a kind of a "homing system", it constantly analyses the entire visual field and decides to direct the gaze towards a new target three times per second on average. It has been calculated that our visual system chooses the target, coordinates the time and determines the spatial parameters of movement 170000 times per day and 5 billion times in a lifetime. Therefore the eye movements are very important for the understanding of human perception. Non-pathological eye movements may be divided into convergent eye movements, tremors – slight oscillations of the eye, drifts, microsaccades, optokinetic movements, following and rapid eye movements (saccades). Apart from those, we can also distinguish fixations, often treated as a separate physiological mechanism and in reality made of small movements called intra-fixation movements, i.e. of the tremor, microsaccades and the drift. Although, as determined by physiology, fixations are in fact movements as well, they are interpreted as fixing the gaze on a particular fragment of the view (a static process by nature), which is by all means justified, as small movements serve the purpose of broadening the precise visual field – as one of the compensation mechanisms.

Observing the tremor of the eye one may notice another of its characteristic features, which is discernible in both eyes. It is movements of approximate frequency of 90 Hz which, due to the critical flicker frequency between 25 and 50 Hz depending on one's psychophysical condition (causing the fusion of images changing with greater frequency), are not subjectively perceived. The role of tremor remains unclear. Some researchers link it to the constant activation of visual neurones (S. Martinez-Conde/S. L. Macknik/D. Hubel 2004). Others write that it may result from the imprecise muscle control of the eye (K. Holmqvist et al. 2011).

Drift is a slow movement of the eye focus away from the fixation point. The role of the drift is to prevent adaptation, that is the decreased sensitivity of the receptor under the influence of a steady stimulus (W. Budohoska/A. Grabowska 1995). Adaptation causes our vision not to be distorted by the shadows cast by blood vessels in the eyeball, as they always fall onto the same spot on the retina (R. Sekuler/R. Blake 1994). As the research quoted by those authors proves, the experimental elimination of slight movements leads to the loss of sight. The role of drift, just like the role of tremor, has not been entirely explained. According to S. Martinez-Conde et al. (2004), drift may have a compensatory role, that is may correct the gaze fixation point when the distortions resulting from the lack of stability of the visual system cause loss of visual acuity. Drift is a mechanism controlled by the central nervous system; as the quoted research indicates, it is distorted in patients with brain stem injury.

Microsaccades, that is small, fast, jerk-like movements, are a mechanism which serves the purpose of returning the gaze to the fixation point (correctional function resulting from small eye movements). Due to the slight instability of the visual system it is necessary for the proper vision to have a mechanism which would allow to refocus the gaze on the observed object. It has also been reported that microsaccades are relevant to the perception of colour shades (S. Martinez-Conde/S. L. Macknik/D. Hubel 2004).

Another type of movement is convergence eye movement. This phenomenon occurs in both eyes at the same time and, thanks to the constriction of the extraocular muscles, directs the visual axis towards one point (movement towards the anterior median line). The purpose of this movement is to place the image of the observed object at the same part of the retina, namely on the fovea. This mechanism is used by the nervous system to measure the depth and is its only absolute indicator. Because the angle differences between the more distant objects are too small to detect, this system is only effective when looking from the distance of no more than 5 metres (V. E. Cavallo/A. S. Cohen 2001). Although moving the object away from the eye is also connected with the change in accommodation (adjusting the focal length of the eye in order to obtain a sharp image), a number of surveys have shown that only convergence gives any clue as to distance estimation (M. W. Levine 2000).

The next type of movement is the saccadic eye movement, which is made three times per second on average. It is related to the amount of time necessary to recognise the object in the fixation point and to plan another movement. In experimental conditions the time between two consecutive saccades may be reduced to approximately 70 milliseconds, as long as the task requires a predetermined sequence of eye movements (E. M. Van Loon/I. Th. C. Hooge/A.V. Van den Berg 2002). Saccades are controlled by the processes occurring in several structures of the nervous system (cf. M. I. Posner/M. E. Raichle 1993). The first element of this process is shifting attention. This means that a fragment of the visual field analysed so far loses its highest priority and is replaced by another visual field. Disengaging attention (that is ending the cognitive processing) from the original target is carried out by the parietal cortex structure (Ch. M. Thiel/K. Ziles/G. R. Fink 2004). The disengagement of attention may be omitted – sometimes the eye movement is made when the visual attention in not engaged (B. Fischer/H. Weber 1993, T. Marek/M. Fąfrowicz 1995, J. Pratt/

C. M. Lajonchere/R. A. Abrams 2006). The frontal lobe structures, on the other hand, are responsible for establishing the moment of eye movement, as well as for the conscious control over its direction. The research quoted by Ch. M. Thiel et al. (2004) indicates the areas located bilaterally of the subparietal sulcus region. The sudden appearance of a new stimulus activates in turn the right temporoparietal junction areas. The ultimate centre of the eye movement, which integrates the signals coming from the areas mentioned, are the superior colliculi (S. P. Liversedge/J. M. Findlay 2000). They transmit the signal further to the brain stem, which coordinates the muscles rotating the eyeball (T. Marek/ M. Fąfrowicz 1995). Also worth noting is a tremendously important phenomenon which occurs after the movement is made, referred to as the inhibition of return. This mechanism prevents the return of the gaze to the previously fixed location, thus serving to facilitate exploration of the visual field. Where this mechanism is located has not been fully explained. There exists a range of empirical data which confirms its connection with the visual areas within the occipital cortex, temporal lobe cortex and parietal lobe cortex (A. R. Mayer/J. M. Dorflinger/S. M. Rao/M. Seidenberg 2004).

Depending on the presence (or absence) of individual components of the eye movement, the following saccades are distinguished: slow, fast and express saccades (B. Fischer/B. Breitmeyer 1987, B. Fischer/S. Gezeck/W. Huber 1995, T. Marek/M. Fąfrowicz 1995). Slow saccades occur over 200 ms from stimulus exposure. These movements engage saccadic mechanisms, that is attention shifts, voluntary control (or its potential presence), calculation of movement parameters and the movement itself. Fast saccades are performed when the attention is disengaged (i.e. no information from the fixation point is being taken at the time). This type of movement may be intentionally stopped, however its direction is determined by stimuli. Its response time varies from 140 to 200 ms. Express saccades are fully reflexive in nature, are performed under 140 ms and follow the direction indicated by automatisms (B. Fischer/H. Weber 1993).

Among intentional saccadic eye movements are saccades and smooth pursuit eye movements. These movements determine the active search for new information. Saccades are believed to be the fastest movements our bodies can perform and usually do not last longer than 80 ms. Saccades normally occur between two fixation points, however they may sometimes form a curve (scanpath). Smooth pursuit movements have similar properties to saccades. The smooth pursuit eye movements occur when a moving object appears in the field of vision. Saccades may appear when observing a white piece of paper (without a stimulus).

The role of smooth pursuit eye movements is to follow a moving object while the head remains relatively immobile. Brain centres responsible for initiating and maintaining smooth pursuit movements block the saccadic eye movements (J. Ross/M. C. Morrone/D. C. Burr 1997). Tracking an object in natural conditions usually also requires a head movement, as well as correction saccades when the object moves away from the fixation point, therefore the mechanisms for coordination of these movements are complex and their effectiveness determines how precise the perception of moving objects is (K. Srihasam/D. Bullock/S. Grossberg 2007). Although traditionally the processes of visual attention have rather been linked to the saccadic eye movements, currently more and more often the role of attention mechanisms in initiating and maintaining the smooth pursuit movements is highlighted (B. Khurana/E. Kowler 1987). In experimental research S. B. Hutton and D. Tegally (2005) proved that the parameters for smooth pursuit movements, such as speed and spatial accuracy, are weakened by performing other tasks which require attention. The smooth pursuit eye movements are not therefore, according to the authors, only dependent on simple neural mechanisms, but similarly to saccadic eye movements depend on a complex cognitive system.

While discussing eye movements one should mention several mechanisms that ensure the stability of perception. If it were not for them, the necessity of recognizing an image anew after each movement would probably make it impossible to maintain a conscious perception. One of such mechanisms is optokinetic reflex. It compensates for head movements in order to maintain fixation on a selected object. Although it is a reflex that occurs without being consciously controlled, it may be blocked (W. Becker/S. Raab/R. Jurgens 2002). Another mechanism is saccadic suppression. Currently it is assumed that the mechanism of that phenomenon consists in the blocking of certain portions of neurons within superior colliculus of the lamina tecti mesencephali (the roofplate of the mesencephalon formed by the quadrigeminal bodies) that are responsible for vision by other portions responsible for saccadic eye movements (P.H. Lee et al. 2007). It is supposed to counterpart visual disturbances that could be caused by quick movement of the image (several times per second). That means that saccadic suppression implies that the part of the image over which a saccade passes becomes invisible. A typical pre-saccadic suppression causes a lack of vision for 30-40 ms that precede the saccade onset, and a post-saccadic suppression "consumes" 100-120 ms of the image vision. Moving a step further, one may assume that a human being cannot see also for the part of the time when a fixation occurs, which should be taken into account when specifying the precise duration of fixation, or to be more precise, the active fixation of vision (K. Holmqvist et al. 2011). Trans-saccadic integration is currently the least researched mechanism from that group. That mechanism occurs on the level of the visual cortex (I. D. Gilchrist/C. A. Heywood/

J. M. Findlay 2003). It is of the highest significance as each saccade movement basically changes the image of the external world reflected onto our retina, thus our visual system has to as it were analyse once more the individual objects and their features. In light of the data compiled by D. Melcher (2005) one should assume that mechanisms of trans-saccadic integration are based or the cortical representation of the space, and not on the retina images. A meaningful element of trans-saccadic integration is at the same time not only image analysis after a saccade occurs, but chiefly analysis of the previous image (D. A. Gajewski/ J. M. Henderson 2005). A series of experiments has shown that a saccadic movement does not interfere with the perception of elements of an image (S. L. Prime/M. Niemeier/J. D. Crawford 2004). Currently studies are conducted in order to establish the limits of the efficiency of that mechanism. It turns out that regardless of the subjective stability of an image, saccadic movements limit to a degree the capacity of visual memory (S. L. Prime et al. 2007). On the other hand, D. Melcher and M. C. Moronne (2003) have shown that trans-saccadic integration of movement information is possible both when its location after a saccade is related to the spatial or retinal location. It has been proven that trans-saccadic integration is not connected with iconic memory, but numerous new findings (J. M. Findlay/I. D. Gilchrist 2003, D. Melcher 2009) prove that the issue of trans-saccadic integration is not only a matter of a simple compensatory mechanism, but it involves attention and active processing of the image. Research concerning trans-saccadic integration, specifically that using neuroimaging techniques, is currently one of the fastest growing fields of research in perception psychology. Explaining that issue requires approaching visual perception as an active manner of information searching, and not only a passive reflection of the outside world.

Although as recently as 15-20 years ago eye movements were more frequently associated with pure physiology that with higher psychological functions, presently is treated as a precise mapping of the interaction(s) between cognitive processes and external stimuli of a visual nature. Along the same lines, some researchers claim that eyetracking is a window of the mind, thought and sense (L. Holm 2007, P.W. Glimcher, 2003), and that vein of thought is reflected in the book published in 2007 edited by Roger van Gompel et al., entitled *Eye movements – a window to mind and brain*. Clearly, such hypotheses as The Eye-Mind Hypothesis (M. A. Just/P. A. Carpenter 1976) had been formulated much earlier to be at least partially undermined later on (J. R. Anderson/D. Bothell/S. Douglass 2004).

Numerous studies have also been conducted to prove the presence of a neurophysiological bridge between eye movement and cognitive functions. One of them is an experiment based on an anti-saccade task testing the processes of attention, memory and decision-making (S. Everling/B. Fischer 1998, D. S. Zee/A. G. Lasker 2004). One should remember however that we are still unable to draw conclusions concerning specific cognitive processes only on the basis of visual perception. It is said that analyses of findings concerning eye movements as a response to a stimulus situation are inaccurate because one does not take into account the complexity of human reactions, associations and classification of the perceived objects.

As eyetracking was becoming more and more popular and information technology and electronics were evolving, methods of measurement of eye movement developed. Currently used methods include electrooculography, video eyetracking and induction method. There also emerge attempts to use computer-aided video cameras, but the precision of such measurement is limited only to the movement that drives the mouse pointer or writing using a virtual keyboard.

Once the most popular method – electrooculography – uses the recording of the potential difference between the cornea and the retina. Electrodes placed around the eye allow to determine the eye movements on both planes (the horizontal and vertical one) on the basis of the recorded voltages. Being relatively cheap, heaving a high sampling frequency. But this method has though numerous limitations. The first of them is the difficulty to adapt to changing lighting; moreover, physiological processes going on in the skin and the eye may be source of artifacts, that is result deformations. Although nominally the precision of measurement in electrooculography is quite good (about 1 degree), it is useful mainly for measuring large saccades. Another limitation is the necessity to maintain good contact between the electrodes and the skin (with the impedance as low as possible), which may be difficult during longer recording sessions.

The most invasive technique of all has been so far the technique that consists in implementing a mechanical or optical reference point onto the eyeball. It enables a very precise recording (in the induction method, with the precision of 5-10 angular seconds), but considering how invasive it is (it is necessary to insert a foreign body into the eye), it causes discomfort, and the experiment duration should be as short as possible (in most cases, no longer than 30 minutes) (L. R. Young/D. Sheena 1975). One of the most popular methods is the implementation of an induction coil enclosed in a special contact lens and measuring movement in an electromagnetic field.

Photo-oculography and video eyetracking are currently the most often employed techniques of the measurement of eye movement, and for that reason we will focus on them in this chapter. As a part of that method a camera or video camera is directed at the eye recording specific elements of the eyeball in motion (the pupil, corneal reflection, corneal limbus etc.). The eye has numerous reference points that may be used. To increase the precision of measurement an additional source of light is used to lighten the eye. This method yields good time and space resolution results. For the first time it was used in thc so-called *Dodge's photochronograph* around 1903. Originally visible light was used for that purpose, but the necessity of using a very intensive light was aggravating for the subject and it lead to numerous artifacts. Ultraviolet light was used as well, but relatively rarely. Currently manufacturers of eyetrackers resort to infrared rays. The first method in this category (the so-called limbus tracker) is based on the fact that the sclera reflects more light than the cornea, thus, directing a beam of infrared rays at the eye and analysing the amount of reflected light we may determine the position of the eye. Recording is possible then even in absolute darkness. The problem might be blinking, which may cause artifacts by covering the eye with the eyelid as well as small shifts of the eyes in the direction of the centre of the head, and thus a change in the light reflection. Video eyetracking is currently used in the three appliances – a Head Mounted Eyetracking system offering the speed up to 360Hz for one eye (H6, ASL), a remote eye-tracking system up to 500Hz for both eyes (RED500), SensoMotoric Instruments) and a superfast eyetracker that requires head stabilizing but enables measurement up to Hz 2000 for one eye (EyeLink 1000, SR Research). Head mounted eyetrackers, owing to their fixed position with reference to the eyes of the subjects eliminate artifacts that may result from head movements, but they also help to liberate the experiment environment from the subject-monitor dependency. That is why that type of appliance serves often as a mobile system. The camera and a source of infrared light are placed under an eye of the subject slightly above or underneath the eye. In most eyetrackers of that type there is also the so-called scene camera that records the space in front of the subject throughout the experiment. Video material made by the camera is used during the analysis – it serves as a rcference image for results visualisation. Up to 2011, scene cameras had used a 640x480 resolution, but in 2011 the first commercial head mounted eyetracker with a scene camera using 1280x960 resolution was launched into the market. Anyone who has ever analysed a material recorded by a head mounted eyetracker will definitely appreciate that technological advancement. In recent years, owing to technological progress and miniaturisation of electronic components, there are glasses available on the market with an embedded eye-tracking system linked to a small recording device or laptop. The speed of the systems has so far been low, but their manufacturers are striving to increase it. In 2011, two interesting systems emerged used in eyeglasses by Tobii and SensoMotoric Instruments (SMI). They are interesting for several reasons – Tobii has developed a special system of active markers which – having been placed in the experimental environment – communicate with the eyetracker during the experiment. Thanks to that arrangement, it is possible to automatically trace the areas of interest during the analysis. The Tobii eyeglasses monitor one eye and work at the speed of 30Hz. While writing the present chapter, we did not found any information regarding their precision of measurement. As regards SMI, it has developed software for semi-automatic aggregation of data and determination of dynamic areas of interest without the necessity of applying markets, whose most important feature (in the authors' view) is the binocular measurement that can compensate for parallax. The SMI eyeglasses work at the speed of 30 Hz for each eye with a maximum measurement deviation of 0.5 degree and spatial resolution of 0.1 degree. Remote eyetrackers use camera and infrared diodes usually positioned above or below the source of stimulus (in most cases, the computer screen to which an eye-tracking interface is attached). Most manufacturers make it possible to use the eyetracker also with other sources of stimuli, such as an OHP screen or TV using a special leg attached to the interface. Remote eyetrackers are sensitive to head movements and if the subject is not willing to cooperate, they must be calibrated every dozen of minutes or so. Nonetheless, all in all, they are the most comfortable and simplest appliances to use. Remote eyetrackers work at the speed of 30-500Hz using one- or two-eyed measurement. Spatial resolution specified by the manufacturers varies from 0.1 to over 1. The last category of eyetrackers covers ultrafast appliances with an eye-tracking interface positioned at the stimulus source or close to the eyes of the subject. They also require a special tower-mounted support frame in which the head of the subject is immobilised. Owing to this element head movements can be eliminated and consequently artifacts resulting from those. Although in theory systems faster than 200Hz can be used to record microsaccades, in practice such experiments are conducted using such ultrafast systems as above-mentioned (S. Martinez-Conde et al. 2009).

It is also worth mentioning that along with increasing interest in functional magnetic resonance imaging of the brain (fMRI), more and more appliances monitoring eye movements emerge into the market that may be used in a magnetic field. Video eyetrackers that offer recording a stimulus and superimposing the image of eye movements are still quite slow; most of them can record images at 50-60 Hz). Their precision varies depending on the type of eyetracker and its manufacturer.

We are aware of numerous simplifications used in this chapter, so any reader interested in the present part of it who wish to expand their knowledge of technology used for eye-tracking research, is encouraged to refer to L.R. Young and D. Sheena (1975), or contemporary publications such as A. Duchowski

(2007), K. Holmqvist et al. (2011) as well as an extremely interesting survey of eye-tracking research authored by N. Wade and B.W. Tatler (2005).

While preparing for an eye-tracking test not only do we have to select our tool, but also match it with an appropriate room and be aware of factors that may influence the quality of results. Clearly there does not exist a single appropriate solution. Test conditions vary depending on the type of experiment – whether it will be conducted outside a laboratory, whether a mobile eyetracker will be used, whether it will be conducted in dedicated rooms – in such cases usually remote eyetrackers and ultrafast eyetrackers will be used (jointly they are referred to by some researchers as table-mounted eyetrackers).

In the first variant we have an opportunity to map (or use) natural or near-natural conditions, which has become more significant in recent years. Simultaneously, in this type of test it is hard to control the experiment conditions which may influence its result. However, since modern mobile systems were made available to researchers, more and more often we can read about projects conducted with participation of athletes, about workstation ergonomic tests, road safety etc. Costs related to distractors or lack of full control of test conditions are counterbalanced by the benefits from the natural conditions of the experiment. This factor is essential when we plan to carry out group analyses of the experiment complete result as it may turn out impossible. Another key element is conditions outside of the buildings – for eye-tracking tests, the sun is the most prominent distractor as the intensity of infrared light in such conditions may outdo significantly the intensity of light emitted by the eyetracker. In such conditions, the researcher will obtain no measurement result as corneal reflection analysis will not be possible.

In tests conducted in a laboratory conditions and distracting factors may vary depending on whether eyetracking is to be the only method we employ or just an element of the experiment, whether the test is carried out in front of a screen or whether it is, for instance, a test in a flight simulator. In any configurations it is important to separate the test operator from the room where the test is conducted. We have often observed the impact of the presence of other persons on the calibration and then result quality. Obviously in usability tests one frequently encounters a situation in which the experiment operator sits near the subject; however, it is justified by the methodology. In most cases laboratories are designed in such a manner that the control room and test room are divided by a wall allowing the latter to be relatively soundproof. For monitoring there are one-way mirrors and an audio system for communication between the rooms. The eyetracker screen is cloned on the external screen placed in the control room. Taking into account fast development of video technology laboratories begin to use high resolution cameras that offer more possibilities than the one-way mirror and simultaneously record the subject and the experiment situation. Cameras are a proven tool also when in one laboratory there are several rooms of simultaneous tests with one control room.

As most eyetrackers that are currently used employ infrared light, one should minimize exposition to sunlight especially if its rays were to reach the eyetracker or the subject's face directly. A recommended type of lighting is fluorescent lamps because they emit a minimal amount of infrared light and considering their frequency. In video eyetracking one should avoid completely dark rooms as in such conditions the pupil becomes so big, that the appliances find it difficult to identify its position. One should also make sure there is a well-stabilised desk on which the eyetracker will be placed as well as guarantee that a mouse and keyboard are positioned on an independent surface so that vibrations that might influence the eyetracker are minimised.

Irrespective of whether we use a head-mounted or table-mounted system during the test we may face some other factors which – if not controlled – may make the measurement impossible or disturb the test results. K. Holmqvist et al. (2011) have classed them into four groups: 1. covering too large a surface of the eyeball, physiologically caused by a dropping eyelid, and functionally – for instance by laughter. 2. Interferences caused by makeup, especially mascara worn on the eyelashes, eyeglasses, contact lenses or dry eyes; 3. Interferences arising from bi-focal eyeglasses; 4. eye image loss caused by head movement.

Although eye movements are linked to brain processes, on the executive level they are effects of purely physiological reactions. Eyes are moved by six muscles which are activated in groups in practically every movement of the eye. Extraocular muscles are controlled by three cranial nerves whose nuclei are linked to other nerves. That guarantees cooperation not only of individual elements of the visual system but it also facilitates adjusting eye movement to reactions of other senses. What is more, an optic nerve is linked to the eye; it is a part of the optic tract through which electric signals reach optic areas in the visual cortex. In order for visual stimuli to be recorded by the brain, they must come the pathway starting from the pupil, passing through the lens only to finally stimulate cone cells and rod cells in the retina in the form of an inverted image. Photoreceptors in the retina are supposed to convert the perceived image into an electric signal. The fovea in the retina offers the best resolution of image recording. It may be found precisely on the horizontal axis of the eye and it covers less than 2° of the field of view. The visual element on which we focus our gaze is mapped onto this part of the retina, hence human beings have such a small span of sharp vision. As a result it is necessary to record the centre of the pupil in order to assess the fixation point. Additionally, another important component for eye position assessment is the cornea, and to be more precise –

the corneal reflection. Contemporary eye-tracking systems based on video technology use a source of infrared light and record its reflection on the cornea and/or lens according to the Purkinje image theory as currently recording all Purkinje images poses little difficulty. The images are reflections of light from the elements of the eye. There are at least four reflections of this type. The first Purkinje image (P1) is a reflection from the outer surface of the cornea. The other image (P2) is a reflection on the inner surface of the cornea. The third image (P3) is a reflection from the anterior surface of the lens and the last image (P4) is a reflection from the posterior surface of the lens. Assessing the position of a reflection with reference to the centre of the pupil facilitates a precise recording of the eye movement.

In order to realise how complicated the process of managing the visual system is one should know that processes of visual perception involve a large part of the brain. Among other things, this pertains to the frontal eye field that generates conjugate eye movements located in the premotoric cortex within the middle frontal gyrus and a lateral part of the precentral sulcus (a structure controlling saccadic movements but also related to fixations), the medial longitudinal fasciculus (as a structure that links the nuclei of oculomotoric nerves), the vestibular nuclei and reticular formation (optical areas in the midbrain that ensure among others the appropriate operation of the visual system during head movements, supervising vergent movements etc.), posterior oculomotor field located in the paretial lobe cortex (the source of reflex saccades), dorsolateral prefrontal cortex (voluntary control of saccades). This structure is an essential substrate of decision processes that divide elements of the perception field into these which should and should not or are not worth involving a reaction in a given situation (Leśniak, 2008). Supervision of the cortex of more complex free saccadic movements requires involving additional structures such as an additional movement fields responsible for learning a sequence of saccades, but also for fixation movements (R. J. Leigh/D. S. Zee 2006). On the other hand, basal ganglia are involved in supervision of brainstem areas, and through that, they play a role of intentional inhibiting and stimulating eye movement. The area where the temporal lobe, parietal lobe and occipital lobe meet is associated with control of pursuit movements. Readers interested in functional anatomy of the brain falling within the scope of this topic are referred to the following source: G. Avanzini/F. Villani 1994, N. Carter/D. S. Zee 1997, R. J. Leigh/D. S. Zee 2006, M. Leśniak 2008.

The information presented so far in this chapter has shown what complicated processes have impact on eye movements and their research. In spite of that eyetracking has already been used in most areas of life and science. Eyetrackers have flown on NASA missions but also with pilots of passenger and military aircraft. Disabled persons use eyetrackers to communicate with others or to operate a computer. Research concerning processes behind eye movement has involved animals but also humans from every age group. Eyetrackers are used in linguistics, but also in psychology, neurology or law. A significant portion of current research is used to decide what type of advertisement is more convincing and understandable or whether websites are functional and well-designed. In this part of the chapter we will focus on a review of research using eye-tracking systems.

Similarly as in the case of numerous behavioural studies, when it comes to eye movement research it is very difficult to determine when it was initiated. N. Wade and B.W. Tatler (2005), who were seeking the first mentions of eye research in available publications, have proven that eye movements have fascinated researchers from time immemorial. Nonetheless, it is common belief that first mentions of eye movements be found in Du Laurens' work in 1596. According to Boring (1942) it is the monograph of Johannes Muller published in 1826 that described for the first time fully-fledged eye-tracking research (N. Wade/B. W. Tatler 2005). The other founding father of eye-tracking research appears to have been Charles Bell, who in his work of 1823 presented findings of research concerning active and passive eye movements as a reaction to visual stimuli and paid attention to proprioception (which he then referred to as muscle sense). One should not forget either the work by Jan Evangelista Purkinje, even though he raised a broader variety of topics – mainly from the field of physiology. Any works written earlier than the above mentioned and many published afterwards concentrate rather on optics, physiology and eye morphology or extraocular muscles, that is physical aspects of eyeball movements than on cognitive processes behind the movement.

The contemporary research concentrates mostly on the relationship between the eye and the brain, or more precisely – on the cognitive processes behind the eye movement, recording at the same time the number of fixations, their duration, the saccades and scan paths, but using state-of-the-art technologies it also correlates these results with response time, "hitting" the target, or the mistakes made. Before that only individual experiments of this kind were conducted, which is accurately described by K. Rayner (1998). Rayner divides the output of eye-tracking research in experimental psychology to date into three stages. The first was begun by Javal, who conducted research into text perception from 1879 until roughly 1920. The second stage, in which initially the same topic was explored, was later (that is approximately until 1950's) characterised by a limited number of studies. One of the more important studies of that era was the eye movement measurements carried out by Buswell (K. Rayner 1998). He showed 55 pieces of art to 200 subjects, manipulating the task instructions given. In his conclusion he stated that “Eye movements are unconscious adjustments to the demands of attention” (A. Duchowski 2007).

Still in the second stage of the eye tracking studies according to Rayner, similar research was repeated by A.L. Yarbus (1967). He referred in it to the visual processes occurring when watching simple and complex stimuli (including texts), moving objects, or optical illusions. Yarbus pointed out the existence of a repetitive component in the perception processes of the target object also taking into account such processes as the visual assessment of proportions, evaluation of length, comparison of areas, etc. He proved that the human eye, both voluntarily and involuntarily, focuses on those objects or their elements which may carry information essential for performing the task. One may contend (after Yarbus) that how long the eyes stay on a given fragment of the image indicates how much important and essential information it carries. The order and duration of individual fixations may help to determine the thought processes (analysis). The third era – the most effective one – begins in mid-1970's. The renaissance of eye-tracking research was begun by the introduction of new technologies to track eye movement – more precise and easy to use – and their development was facilitated by the introduction of computers allowing to gather data more effectively or analyse them faster.

One of the most explored topics was the processes of visual perception, or more precisely visual attention. In the course of experiments in which those processes were investigated a number of important mechanisms were observed. One of them is saccadic suppression already discussed above. It is worth repeating that this phenomenon consists in decreasing the responsiveness of the visual system to stimuli during fast eye movements.

Another mechanism is the relatively comparable duration of fixation, or the length of saccade, for a given type of stimulus perceived. For silent reading, scanning or e.g. writing the length of saccades varies from 1 up to even 5°; similarly does the mean fixation duration - it varies, however in many studies for a particular stimulus remains the same (cf. S. G. Abrams /B. L. Zubel 1972, R. A. Abrams/D. E. Meyer/S. Kornblum 1989). Of course, the length of saccades or the fixation duration is influenced by more factors than only the type of stimulus, and these could be purely physiological mechanisms, but also cognitive processes (e.g. accessing memory stores, attention, etc.). Another mechanism which supports the claim that eye movements are closely related to executive processes is latency of saccadic movements, that is the time between the onset of the stimulus and initiation of eye movement. Ususally the latency time is over 150 ms, even in a situation where we are dealing with such automatic processes as reading a text. During tens of years of research into the latency of saccades a number of essential facts was found (after: K. Rayner

1998). Among other things independent decision-making processes responsible for eye movement programming were discovered. It has also been proved that cognitive processes may increase latency (H. Deubel, 1995). A corelation between the length of latency and precise location of the visual target was found (Nazir and Jacobs, 1991). It was verified that giving instructions to direct attention when performing the task also increases latency (C. Coëffe/ J. K. O'Regan 1987, E. Kowler/E. Blaser 1995). However, disappearance of the target before attention is shifted to it decreases latency (A. Kingstone/ R. M. Klein 1993; L. E. Ross/S. M. Ross 1980, 1981).

In the world of eye-tracking research a lot of attention is paid to reading processes. One of the most widely quoted publications in eye tracking is a collection of theories and review of studies in this area developed by K. Rayner (1998). It is no exaggeration to say that eye movements directly reflect the processes of language processing. The subject that raises the most interest in this field is understanding of the relationship between text comprehension and eye movement. Many studies, if not all of them, have proved that comprehension of a sentence is almost instantaneous, however we still do not know the individual components which coordinate this process. So far at least several models of eye movement control in the reading process have been devised. In order to become acquainted with one of the most popular and comprehensive models refer to the publication on E-Z Reader model by Reichle, Pallatsek, Fisher and Rayner (see E. D. Reichle et al. 1998 for more details).

The reading process studies have revealed several important mechanisms. One of the most important mechanisms is the duration of fixation on a word (and often shortening of saccades that is conditioned by that mechanism,). Reading aloud or concentrating on the text that one is listening to produces longer fixations on words than silent reading. M. A. Just and P. A. Carpenter (1980) recorded longer fixations on less common words than on words that are used more frequently. Further research into this phenomenon revealed that this effect fades with a word's high frequency of use in a short text fragment, so when seen for the third time, there is no difference in the fixation duration between the same rare word and high frequency words (Ch. Clifton/A. Staub/ K. Rayner 2007). This effect can also be observed in frequent words, but is not as pronounced. A similar rule applies to word familiarity – the more familiar the word to the reader, the shorter the fixation (R. Chaffin/R. K. Morris/R. E. Seely 2001). The duration of fixation on a word is also influenced by word predictability from the preceding context. Such effect was described by S. F. Ehrlich/K. Rayner (1981), and the following research yielded a further conclusion that predictability also causes the highly predictable words to be more often skipped during reading (K. Rayner/A. D. Well 1996). These factors are directly linked to the effect caused by the processing of a word with respect to the age in which we acquired it. The later we acquired the word, the slower we process it, and therefore the longer the fixation of the word (B. J. Juhasz 2005). The situation is similar with the word complexity – the higher the number of morphemes, the longer it is registered by the visual system (J. Hyönä/ A. Pollatsek 1998). Considering the subject matter of this book, those interested in this topic are further referred to its later chapters, to the book edited by K. Rayner (1992) and the book edited by van Gompel et al. (2007).

Just as often reviewing the literature of the topic reveals experiments regarding scene perception. While some models of visual perception in reading are already known, there are no such studies for the strategies employed scene perception processes. The scanpaths in reading are strictly defined, yet in scene perception the scanpaths may differ even for the same or a similar image. A mere change of task can be the factor influencing the process of image perception. However, there is a number of definite dependencies or rules. As has been said so far, many researchers (A.L. Yarbus as probably the first one, 1967) proved that fixations on an element of the image are closely related to the task performed and most often result from the need to obtain information carried by this element. The next fact drawn from the studies is that the image recognition performance increases with increasing number of fixations (G. R. Loftus, 1981). Probably the basic information regarding a scene is registered and processed basing on the first fixation, however this information is imprecise considering the physiological constraints of vision perception (vision acuity only within a small area around the point of fixation) (see K. Rayner, A. Pollatsek 1992). If a given element of the image is important, we may be positive that in the course of the image perception the fixations will be precisely directed at that element. From the perspective of analysing the scene perception processes equally important are not only the number and duration of fixations, but also their order. Many studies have noted the likeness of the effect produced by the duration of fixation on an element to the duration of fixation on a word. The element which is contextually consistent with the scene and is recognizable shortens the fixation duration (J. M. Henderson/A. Hollingworth 1998, K. Rayner 1998).

Marketing research and website usability testing are also undergoing quite a dynamic development, however the vast majority of companies are not interested in publishing the results of their studies or describing the methodology applied. One of very few studies available to readers is a work published on the Nielsen Norman Group website, which describes the usability testing methodology with the use of eye tracking (K. Pernice/J. Nielsen 2009). The use of eye tracking in marketing research is mostly valued for its identification of attention areas – elements which attract the attention of a potential customer, clarity of advertising message, brand visibility in marketing materials or product packaging, etc. Such research is conducted in laboratories with the use of a monitor, television set or a projector, but the highest value is attached to those studies which are conducted in the natural environment – in the service space or in the street.

As has already been mentioned in this chapter several times – eye-tracking research has been experiencing a renaissance for quite some time now (at least since 1980's). It has presently become such a broad topic that one chapter, or even one comprehensive book will never be exhaustive enough to fully reveal all its secrets. This is why at every important point we have tried to indicate further reading to expand the information provided in this chapter. Those readers who are interested in the topic of eye tracking may wish to refer to those titles as we wish they could explore this field with a passion much like ours.

References

Abrams, S. G./ B. L. Zubel (1972): *Some temporal characteristics of information processing during reading*. In: Reading Research Quarterly. 12. 41–51.

Abrams, R. A./ D. E. Meyer/ S. Kornblum (1989): *Speed and accuracy of saccadic eye movements: Characteristics of impluse variability in the oculomotor system.* In: Journal of Experimental Psychology: Human Perception and Performance. 15. 529–543.

Anderson, J. R./ D. Bothell/ S. Douglass (2004): *Eye Movements Do Not Reflect Retrieval Processes. Limits of the Eye–Mind Hypothesis*. In: Psychological Science. 15(4). 225–231.

Avanzini, G / F. Villani (1994): *Ocular movements*. In: Current Opinion in Neurology. 7. 74–80.

Becker, W./ S. Raab/ R. Jurgens (2002): *Circular vection during voluntary suppression of optokinetic reflex*. In: Experimental Brain Research. 144. 554–557.

Budohoska, W./ A. Grabowska (1995): *Procesy percepcji*. In: T. Tomaszewski (ed.), Psychologia ogólna. Warszawa. 9–90.

Carter, N./ D. S. Zee (1997): *The anatomical localization of saccades using functional imaging studies and transcranial magnetic stimulation*. In: Current Opinion in Neurology. 10. 10–17.

Cavallo, V. E./ A. S. Cohen (2001): *Perception*. In: P.E. Baronet (ed.), Traffic Psychology Today. Dordrecht.

Chaffin, R./ R. K. Morris/ R. E. Seely (2001): *Learning new word meanings from context: A study of eye movements*. In: Journal of Experimental Psychology: Learning, Memory and Cognition. 27. 225–235.

Clifton, Ch./ A. Staub/ K. Rayner (2007): *Eye Movements In Reading Words And Sentences*. In: R. P. G. Van Gompel/ M. H. Fischer/ W. S. Murray/ R. L. Hill (eds), Eye Movements: A Window on Mind and Brain. Elsewier. 341–372.

Coëffe, C./ J. K. O'Regan (1987): *Reducing the influence of nontarget stimuli on saccade accuracy: Predictability and latency effects*. In: Vision Research. 27. 227–240.

Deubel, H. (1995): *Separate addaptive mechanisms for the control of reactive and volitional saccadic eye movements*. In: Vision Research. 35. 3529–3540.

Duchowski, A. T. (2007): *Eye Tracking Methodology. Theory and Practice*. London.

Ehrlich, S. F./ K. Rayner (1981): *Contextual effects on word perception and eye movements during reading*. In: Journal of Verbal Learning and Verbal Behavior. 20. 641–655.

Everling, S./ B. Fischer (1998): *The antisaccade a review of basic research and clinical studies*. In: Neuropsychologia. 36(9). 885–899.

Findlay, J. M./ I. D. Gilchrist (2003): *Active Vision: The Psychology of Looking and Seeing*. Oxford.

Fischer, B./ B. Breitmeyer (1987): *Mechanisms of visual attention revealed by saccadic eye movements*. Neuropsychologia. 25.73–83.

Fischer, B./ H. Weber (1993): *Express saccades and visual attention*. In: Behavioral and Brain Sciences. 16. 553–610.

Fischer, B./ S. Gezeck/ W. Huber (1995): *The three loop model: a neural network for the generation of saccadic reaction times*. In: Biological Cybernetics. 72. 185–196.

Gajewski, D. A./ J. M. Henderson (2005): *The role of saccade targeting and in the transsacadic integration of object types and tokens*. In: Journal of Experimental Psychology: Human Perception and Performance. 31. 820–830.

Gilchrist, I. D./ C. A. Heywood/ J. M. Findlay (2003): *Visual sensitivity in search tasks depends on the response requirement*. In: Spatial Vision. 16. 277–293.

Glimcher, P. W. (2003) *The neurobiology of visual–saccadic decision making*. In: Annual Review of Neuroscience. 26. 133–179.

Van Gompel, R. P. G./ M. H. Fischer/ W. S. Murray/ R. L. Hill (2007): *Eye Movements: A Window on Mind and Brain*. Elsevier.

Henderson, J. M./ A. Hollingworth (1998): *Eye Movements During Scene Viewing: An Overview*. In: G. Underwood (ed.), Eye Guidance in Reading and Scene Perception. Elsevier. 269–294.

Holm, L. (2007): *Predictive eyes recede retrieval. Visual recognition as hypothesis testing*. Department of Psychology, Umea University Sweden. (PhD Thesis). Umea

Holmqvist, K./ M. Nyström/ R. Andersson/ R. Dewhurst/ H. Jarodzka/ J. van de Weijer (2011): *Eye Tracking: A comprehensive guide to methods and measures*. Oxford.

Hutton, S.B./ D. Tegally (2005): *The effects of dividing attention on smooth pursuit eye movements*. In: Experimental Brain Research. 163. 306–313.

Hyönä, J./ A. Pollatsek (1998): *Reading Finnish compound words: Eye fixations are affected by component morphemes*. In: Journal of Experimental Psychology: Human Perception and Performance. 24. 1612–1627.

Juhasz, B. J. (2005): *Age–of–acquisition effects in word and picture processing*. In: Psychological Bulletin. 13. 684–712.

Just, M. A./ P. A. Carpenter (1976): *Eye fixations and cognitive processes*. In: Cognitive Psychology. 8. 441–480.

Just, M. A./ P. A. Carpenter (1980): *A theory of reading: from eye fixation to comprehension*. In: Psychological Review. 87. 329–354.

Khurana, B./ E. Kowler (1987): *Shared attentional control of smooth eye movement and perception*. In: Vision Research. 27. 1603–1618.

Kingstone, A./ R. M. Klein (1993): *Visual offset facilitates saccade latency: Does pre–disengagement of attention mediate the gap effect?* In: Journal of Experimental Psychology: Human Perception and Performance. 19. 251–265.

Kowler, E./ E. Blaser (1995): *The accuracy and precision of saccades to small and larger targets*. In: Vision Research. 35. 1741–1754.

Lee, P. H./ T. Sooksawate/ Y. Yanagawa/ K. Isa/ T. Isa/ W. C. Hall (2007): *Idenity of a pathway for saccadic suppression*. In: Proceedings of National Academy of Science. 104. 6824–6827.

Leigh, R. J./ D. S. Zee (2006): *The neurology of eye movements*. Oxford.

Leśniak, M. (2008): *Disorders of the eye movement control in Wilson's disease*. Institute of Psychiatry and Neurology. Warszawa (PhD Thesis).

Levine, M.W. (2000): *Fundamentals of Sensation and Perception*. Oxford.

Liversedge, S. P./ J. M. Findlay (2000): *Saccadic eye movements and cognition*. In: Trends In Cognitive Sciences. 1. 6–14.

Loftus, G. R. (1981): *Tachistoscopic Simulations of Eye Fixations on Pictures*. In: Journal of Experimental Psychology: Human Learning and Memory. 7(5). 369–376.

Van Loon, E. M./ I. Th. C. Hooge/ A. V. Van den Berg (2002): *The timing of sequences of saccades in visual search*. In: Proceedings of the Royal Society of London. 269.

Marek, T./ M. Fąfrowicz (1995): *Neuropsychologiczne mechanizmy procesu przenoszenia uwagi wzrokowej*. In: Kolokwia Psychologiczne. 3. 69–86.

Martinez-Conde, S./ S. L. Macknik/ D. Hubel (2004): *The role of fixational eye movements in visual perception*. In: Nature Reviews Neuroscience. 4. 229–240.

Martinez-Conde, S./ S. L. Macknik/ X. G. Troncoso/ D. H. Hubel (2009): *Microsaccades: a neurophysiological analysis*. In: Trends in Neurosciences. 32(9). 463–475.

Mayer A. R./ J. M. Dorflinger/ S. M. Rao/ M. Seidenberg (2004): *Neural networks underlying endogenous and exogenous visual–spatial orienting*. In: NeuroImage. 23. 534–541.

Melcher, D./ M.C. Moronne (2003): *Spatiotopic temporal integration of visual motion across saccadic eye movements*. In: Nature Neuroscience. 8. 877–881.

Melcher, D. (2005): *Spatiotopic transfer of visual form adaptation across saccadic eye movements*. In: Current Biology. 15. 1745–1748.

Melcher, D. (2009) *Selective attention and the active remapping of object features in trans–saccadic perception*. In: Vision Research. 49. 1249–1255.

Nazir, T. A./ A. M. Jacobs (1991): *The effects of target discriminability and retinal eccentricity on saccade latencies: An analysis in terms of variable–criterion theory*. In: Psychological Research. 53. 281–289.

Pernice, K./ J. Nielsen (2009): *Eyetracking Methodology. How to Conduct and Evaluate Usability Studies Using Eyetracking*. Nielsen Norman Group.

Posner, M.I/ M.E. Raichle (1994): *Images of Mind*. New York.

Pratt, J./ C. M. Lajonchere/ R. A. Abrams (2006): *Attentional modulation of gap effect*. In: Vision Research. 46. 2602–2607.

Prime, S. L. / M. Niemeier/ J. D. Crawford (2004): *Trans– saccadic integration of the orientation and location features of linear objects*. In: Journal of Vision. 8. 742.

Prime, S. L./ L. Tsotsos/ G. P. Keith/ J. D. Crawford (2007): *Visual memory capacity in transsacadic integration*. In: Experimental Brain Reearch. 180. 609–628.

Rayner, K. (ed.) (1992): *Eye Movements and Visual Cognition: Scene Perception and Reading*. New York.

Rayner, K./ A. Pollatsek (1992): *Eye Movements and Scene Perception*. In: Canadian Journal of Psychology. 46(3). 342–376.

Rayner, K./ A. D. Well (1996): *Effects of contextual constraint on eye movements in reading: A further examination*. In: Psychonomic Bulletin & Review. 3. 504–509.

Rayner, K. (1998): *Eye Movements in Reading and Information Processing: 20 Years of Research*. In: Psychological Bulletin. 124(3). 372–422.

Reichle, E. D./ A. Pollatsek/ D. L. Fisher/ K. Rayner (1998): *Toward a Model of Eye Movement Control in Reading*. In: Psychological Review. 105(1). 125–157.

Ross, L. E./ S. M. Ross (1980): *Saccade latency and warning signals: Stimulus onset, offset and change as warning events*. In: Perception & Psychophysics. 27. 251–257.

Ross, S. M./ L. E. Ross (1981): *Saccade latency and warning signals: Effects of auditory and visual offset and onset*. In: Perception & Psychophysics. 29. 429–437.

Ross J./ M. C. Morrone/ D. C. Burr (1997): *Compression of visual space before saccades*. In: Nature. 386(6625). 598–601.

Sekuler, R./ R. Blake (1994): *Perception*. New York.

Srihasam, K./ D. Bullock/ S. Grossberg (2007): *Coordinating saccades and smooth pursuit eye movements during visual tracking and perception of objects moving with variable speeds*. In: Journal of Vision. 6. 908.

Thiel, Ch. M./ K. Ziles/ G. R. Fink (2004): *Cerebral correlates of orienting and reorienting visuospatial attention: an event–related fMRI study*. In: Neuroimage. 21. 318–328.

Wade, N./ B. W. Tatler (2005): *The moving tablet of the eye. The origins of modern eye movement research.* Oxford.

Yarbus, A. L. (1967): *Eye Movements and Vision*. Plenum Press.

Young, L. R./ D. Sheena (1975): *Survey of eye movement recording methods*. In: Behavior research methods, instruments and computers. 7(5). 397–429.

Zee, D. S./ A. G. Lasker (2004): *Antisaccades Probing cognitive flexibility with eye movements*. In: Neurology. 63. 1554.

Eye-Tracking Supported Research Into Sight Translation. Lapsological Conclusions

Monika Płużyczka (University of Warsaw)

Although a relatively young discipline of science, translation studies can already pride itself on its considerable theoretical achievements. These achievements, in particular those concerning the explanation of mental processes involved during translation, have been heavily reliant on hypotheses and assumptions as to what may be happening in the mind of the translator. This is understandable in a situation where the brain of the subject is inaccessible for direct observation. Still, we do have translation products and the ability to research and observe the translation process itself, i.e. the translator's actions. Recent technological advances also enable us to gain an insight into the processes which accompany the process of translation, such as visual perception or even the activity in certain brain regions. Assumptions are formulated more easily when based on empirical facts. Unfortunately, empirical research into translation processes has not yet taken a prominent, dare I say, satisfactory position within translation studies. This would seem the perfect place to express regret over such a situation, as these investigations should be acknowledged as one of the most essential elements in the process of pushing back our borders of cognition (i.e. the limits of our knowledge). They should also be recognized as a major element translating directly or indirectly into the applicative aspect, that is to say, into translodidactic practice[1].

This paper presents selected eye-tracking results carried out within a scientific experiment and the analysis of these results from the lapsological and translodidactic points of view. It also aims to draw attention to the possibilities of applying eye-tracking to the process of translodidactics. I shall demonstrate the challenges of sight translation, and the need for a separate didactic approach to it.

1.

Empirical research into translation studies, carried out since the 1980s, has mainly relied on the data elicited from tests, interviews, questionnaires, and, in order to identify the reasons why students make errors and what motivates them

1 For more details on the term "translodidactics" see Płużyczka 2009a, 2009b, 2009c; 2011c.

to apply particular translation solutions – TAPs[2], i.e. "think aloud protocols". The 1990s saw rapid advances in computer technology and its employment in translation studies research. Research teams making use of the latest computer technology, video recording, screen recording and key logging in translodidactic and translation studies research projects emerged. After the year 2000, eye-tracking (frequently combined with other research methods) was incorporated into research. One of the teams employing eye-tracking (methodology) was the team under professor Susanne Göpferich, at the University of Graz, Austria, involved in the TransComp project. Using a tailored programme called Translog the researchers explored the development of translation competences in 12 subjects over a period of three years. The study population consisted of students with German as their mother tongue – language A, and English as their foreign language – language B. It is worth mentioning that only students with the highest A-level results, good and very good grades in both languages, were selected to participate in the research. 10 professional translators were also invited to join the project. At the end of the project students were asked to translate 10 texts, 5 of which were also translated by each of professional translators. The project was started in October 2007 and aimed to develop methodology and model building in process-oriented translation studies. The texts to be translated contained a number of translation difficulties (lexical, syntactic, pragmatic, culture-specific etc.). The texts were translated using Translog, which registered all the keyboard strokes and mouse activity and the time intervals between them. To guarantee so-called 'ecological validity'[3] the subjects could use the Internet and any other electronic resources. Eye-tracking equipment was also employed in the experiment. During the experiment a subject had either to 'think aloud', that is to concurrently translate the text and to comment on what s/he was doing and why, or to comment on the translation process retrospectively (so-called 'immediate retrospection'). In order to support the retrospection a video recording was played back. Subsequently, the verbal data were transcribed with the use of XML markup; transcripts included information on the use of the Internet and other sources by each individual subject. The TransComp project showed how advances in technology, including eye-tracking, have opened the way for linguistic, translation studies and, most of all, translodidactic research.

2 TAP – think aloud protocols; although the expression "to think aloud" gives this name a highly metaphoric character, I shall continue with using it in this paper as the name is already recognized and deeply rooted in the language of linguistics.

3 Ecological validity – a characteristic of the outcome of the measurement, experiment, research etc. that can refer to real life conditions. In other words, the results have an empirical point of reference in nature.

The last ten years have witnessed the employment of eye-tracking methodology in translation studies and its increasingly widespread use in broadly understood glottodidactics and linguistics. The 'Eye-to-IT' project, as well as many other projects carried out by the Copenhagen Business School may serve as examples. Johannes Gutenberg University in Mainz (Fakultät für Translations-, Sprach- und Kulturwissenschaft – Faculty in Germersheim, with professor Silvia Hansen-Schirra in charge of its eye-tracking laboratory, "houses" numerous projects applying eye-tracking to translation studies and linguistics. Other projects have been carried out by the ATRC (Advanced Translation Research Center) at the University of Saarbrücken. Although eye-tracking research is currently being conducted by professor Max Crocker and his team at Saarland University, it is not limited to just translation processes but encompasses linguistics more generally, while the University of Freiburg supports its investigations with the use of EEG tests. In Poland, eye-tracking research into the mental aspects of the translation process (mostly audio description) is carried out at Adam Mickiewicz University in Poznań by I. Mazur and A. Chmiel. In Warsaw such research is conducted by A. Szarkowska at the University of Warsaw and I. Krejtz at the Warsaw School of Social Sciences and Humanities. A large scale equipment-supported research project, led by professor S. Grucza, Head of the Linguistics of Languages for Specific Purposes Department, has been carried out since 2011 at the Institute of Anthropocentric Linguistics and Culturology at the University of Warsaw. In 2012 a new Eye-tracking Experimental Linguistics Laboratory was established and I took overall charge of it[4].

2.

A pilot study was carried out in April 2011. The study population consisted of 17 subjects: one professional interpreter and 16 students from the Institute of Anthropocentric Linguistics and Culturology. These were third-year students studying Languages for Specific Purposes (6th term out of a six-term BA course). For ten of these students Russian was their B language (first foreign language), for six it was their C language (second foreign language). The professional interpreter was a Russian language interpreter.

The aims of the research were extensive and comprehensive. They were as follows:

1. to analyze the cognitive possibilities of eye-tracking research in translation studies, with the following key questions put forward: what results can be

4 www.lelo.uw.edu.pl

obtained, what do they indicate, what conclusions can be arrived at, to what extent and within what scope is this method of research useful for translation studies (and also for linguistics)? (c.f. M. Płużyczka 2012);
2. to observe how the subjects receive information, how they read, how much time has lapsed from the perception of information to its processing, which information is rendered quickest, which information constitutes a difficulty for them, how wide their peripheral field of vision is, how often re-fixations occur;
3. to arrive at and formulate conclusions concerning the translodidactic relevance of eye-tracking studies – the following questions were asked: (i) What errors do the subjects make in the investigated type of translation and why? (ii) Which elements are fixated on longest, and which elements receive most re-fixations, in other words, what constitutes the greatest difficulty for the subjects? (iii) Are they aware of what constitutes a translation difficulty for them and is there a correlation between their opinion and a long fixation time registered on particular elements?

In the sections to follow, I would like to address the third point, namely the issues that relate to the lapsological and translodidactic aspects of the conducted experiment. I will therefore attempt to answer the question of how subjects deal with sight translation tasks, in other words, I will attempt to formulate answers to the following questions: (a) do the subjects encounter translation difficulties, and if so, of what kind? (b) What translation solutions do they apply? (c) Do translation difficulties result in longer fixations or re-fixations? (d) do the subjects make errors, and if so, what types of errors are they? (e) At what level and where do errors occur most frequently in sight translation?

The study population consisted of two groups of subjects:

Group 1 (13 April 2011): Third-year students, Russian – language C

Name	Sex	Age	Russian as language B (1) language C (2)	Number of years of learning Russian
P1 (Professional translator)	F	32	1	13
P2	F	21	2	4
P3	F	22	2	3
P4	M	25	2	6
P5	M	20	2	6
P6	F	22	2	6
P7	F	21	2	6

Group 2 (14 April 2011): Third-year students, Russian – language B

Name	Sex	Age	Russian as language B (1) language C (2)	Number of years of learning Russian
P8	F	22	1	9
P9	F	22	1	4
P10	F	21	1	6
P11	F	21	1	6
P12	F	22	1	6
P13	F	21	1	7
P14	F	22	1	6
P15	F	21	1	6
P16	F	21	1	12
P17	F	21	1	6

The above tables illustrate that the majority of the students (10) had been studying Russian for 6 years. There are however exceptions, when this period was shorter (3 and 4 years), as well as longer (7 and 12 years). These differences, as the research will prove, will have no bearing on the results of the experiment. The resulting data analysis does not include gender differentiation, as the study group was predominantly female, with only two male subjects.

The eye-tracking research was carried out using a Tobii T120[5] eye tracker. It is a measuring device integrated into a 17" monitor. Eye ball movements are observed with an infrared light scanner located under the monitor. A special camera registers the reflection of the beams in an eye ball (eye movement is measured on the basis of changes in the amount of reflected light), and the collected data is then transferred to a computer to be analyzed and the results delivered. Subjects' behavior and reactions are video recorded too, either with a device integrated into the monitor or a camera attached to it.

The Tobii T120 performs very well in research using printed texts or monitor-based stimuli such as texts (or images). The number 120 refers to the number of Hz, i.e. cycles, in other words, the number of samples (events) per second. In text-based research this measurement is sufficient (250 Hz is possible as well), as the higher number of Hz blurs the picture of all the overlapping gaze plots registered.

5 For the purpose of this research, the eye-tracker was very kindly made available to us by Eyetracking.pl (http://eyetracking.pl).

The device has an inbuilt speaker which allows sound recording, in this case, of the voice of the subjects, a sound signal which constitutes the translated text. Very good head-movement compensation allows interpreters to behave naturally and feel relatively comfortably in front of the screen. Therefore, in an environment very close to a natural testing environment, eye-tracking in experimental situations can deliver, despite subjects' movements, highly accurate and reliable results.

3.

The two three-paragraph source texts, from the domain of economics, constituted the research material. The Russian text contained 182 words (1302 characters with spaces) and referred to the labour market. The Polish text contained 201words (1568 characters with spaces) and referred to changes in the Polish educational system. During the experiment subjects were asked to sight translate a source text into their foreign or mother tongue, depending on the language the text was formulated in. There was an interval of a few minutes between the translation into and out of their mother tongue.

For the purpose of this research the following selection criteria for the research material were adopted:

- The text should not be too complicated, sentences should not be complex and nor should the syntax be too difficult to make translation possible.
- The text should be selected in such a way so as to ensure it contains the following translation difficulties: (a) proper names including names and surnames, (b) abbreviations and acronyms, (c) specialized terms, (d) numerals, (e) metaphors, and (f) collocations and phrases. In selecting the above I drew on the results of an experiment I carried out in 2008 (data material for my PhD dissertation[6]) and selected errors most frequently made by students (depending on their frequency in the text).
- The text should not be saturated with specialized vocabulary, as mastering such vocabulary did not constitute the object of this research. The level of assimilating terms related to a specialized domain, taught during the already completed course was not verified here. Admittedly, the text contained some specific terms, but only those commonly encountered on a daily basis in news reports. The aim was to observe how students approach these terms, whether they can find (or know) their direct equivalents, and if not, what translation techniques they apply.

---

6 Płużyczka M., 2009, *Psycholingwistyczne aspekty dydaktyki translacji tekstów specjalistycznych na materiale rosyjskich tekstów prawnych*), Warszawa, unpublished PhD dissertation.

- The text should contain all the principal parts of speech: adjectives, nouns, verbs, and adverbs. This aims to draw comparisons between parts of speech and present those which have received the longest fixation, and then answer why it was so; are these the areas which students find most difficult?
- The text should be selected so that there is no need for interference (simplification in terms of language and content), so that the principle of authenticity applied in translation didactics may be preserved. The translation process should be as near to the real translation situation as possible.

Even though it was the Polish text and its translation into Russian that constituted the object of my data analysis to give a full insight into the experiment, I am also presenting the Russian text below. The Russian text and its translation into Polish will constitute the object of a separate data analysis.

Text 1: Russian text

The Russian text comes from Russian news agency "Rosbalt-Moscow", the news was broadcast on March 23th, 2011 at 1.18pm[7], in the "Analitics" section. For the purpose of this experiment the text required adaptation, namely, it was considerably shortened. The first three paragraphs with no highly specialized terms or complicated proper names constituted the text to be translated. Its final version runs as follows:

> Оказывается, сегодняшние выпускники вузов начали вполне реалистично смотреть на свою стартовую зарплату! Все мы хорошо помним недавние запросы инфантильных юношей на пороге диплома, сколько по этому поводу было шуток. Как подтвердила руководитель Career.ru, действительно еще пару-тройку лет назад выпускники претендовали в среднем на 60 тыс. рублей в месяц, им давали вдвое меньше, они обижались, и была масса случаев, когда юноша бледный долго и, как правило, тщетно искал доходное место, «плохо начиная жизнь».
>
> Так вот, теперь – совершенно не так. «Спрос и предложение» по части зарплаты, оказывается, практически совпадают, колеблясь вокруг 28-30 тыс. рублей. Зафиксирована и разница между «спросом и предложением»: что-то около 500 рублей, всего-навсего.
>
> Из сегодняшних выпускников, как рассказала Елена Емеленко, легче всего находят работу специалисты по маркетингу и рекламе, PR, IT, а также по кадрам – теперь это все чаще называется HR. Берут людей также в банковский сектор, но молодым экономистам чаще предлагается поработать менеджером по продажам, к чему далеко не все из них готовы. По словам Емеленко, работодатели относительно щедры и обычно предлагают вначале «стажировку», но вполне оплачиваемую и часто приносящую реальное трудоустройство.

---

7 http://www.rosbalt.ru/moscow/2011/03/28/833118.html

Text 2: Polish text

The text, titled "Pay rises for researchers in two years" comes from the TVP Info service, and was broadcast on April 15th, 2011 (at 9.23 pm)[8]. The text underwent more adaptation procedures than the Russian text:

- Some text fragments formulated in indirect speech (quoted expressions) were rewritten into direct speech so that the text was not overfilled with quotations and therefore easier for students to sight translate; the *ad-hoc* character of sight translation does not allow students to get acquainted with the text prior to translation.
- Transformation of indirect speech into direct speech necessitated changes in the word order.
- The names of the programme and TV channel were left out, so as not to extend the duration of sight translation. Students might have found these elements difficult and fixated on them longest.
- Certain words referring to date and time were removed from the text to ensure its universal character and thus not limit it to a narrow time period.
- Paragraph 2 (*Większe nakłady na naukę mamy zapisane w skorygowanym dzisiaj planie finansów do 2014 roku. Dajemy sobie półtora roku na wdrożenie zmian zaproponowanych w ustawach. Potem ruszą podwyżki – powiedziała*) was left out due to its too complex sentence structure and because it was too big a fragment of indirect speech.
- Short quotations at the end of the text were left unaltered to see how the subjects would deal with them.

The final version of the Polish text was as follows:

> Minister Nauki i Szkolnictwa Wyższego profesor Barbara Kudrycka zapowiedziała, że w 2012 roku będzie znaczące dofinansowanie nauki, a podwyżki ruszą najpóźniej w styczniu 2013 roku. Dodała, że podpisane ostatnio przez prezydenta ustawy reformujące system szkolnictwa wyższego doprowadzą do sytuacji, gdzie „student będzie najważniejszym partnerem uczelni".
>
> Prezydent Bronisław Komorowski podpisał ustawy reformujące szkolnictwo wyższe. Do najważniejszych zapisów należy wprowadzenie opłat za drugi kierunek studiów. Ograniczona zostanie też możliwość pracy profesora na kilku uczelniach na raz. Ustawy likwidują też na uczelni stanowisko docenta.
>
> Zdaniem minister nauki, ustawy „ograniczą złe cechy szkolnictwa wyższego". – Każde studia tworzą u absolwentów wartość dodaną. Zależy nam na tym, by ta wartość była jak największa. Świat staje się coraz bardziej konkurencyjny. Mamy fantastycznych młodych ludzi, którzy nie mają kompleksów. Powinni być wykorzystywani do budowy społeczeństwa obywatelskiego w Polsce – wyjaśniła.

---

8 http://tvp.info/informacje/polska/podwyzki-dla-naukowcow-za-dwa-lata/4275578

This is the text that will be researched in this paper. However, let me first briefly introduce the type of translation selected for this experiment.

4.

The technical capabilities of eye-trackers determine, to a certain extent, the type of translation to research. As it turns out, the ultimate research and cognitive possibilities can be linked to eye-tracking supported research into the process of sight translation. This mainly results from the fact that in sight translation the source text takes a written form and is to be rendered orally in the target language. A subject reads a text displayed on the monitor. In the process, the eye-tracker registers his/her eye ball movements, whereas orally produced translation is audio and video recorded.

However, this is not the only reason why I am currently focused on researching sight translation. My interest in this type of translation also results from its unique properties: the synchronicity of visual and auditory stimuli, and its hybrid form where the text is received visually and produced orally, making this seemingly easy and straight forward operation highly difficult. This results in sight translation being difficult to classify and requiring a separate approach within the field of translation studies. As a consequence, it has not received due attention from researchers. It is my view that it is of the utmost necessity that sight translation be subjected to systematic and experimental research, and theoretical description.

Sight translation involves, as mentioned above, rendering the written source language material orally in the target language. The resulting content corresponds to the content of the original written text. Since a translator is expected to reproduce information almost immediately, s/he has very little time to receive the text. This in fact, makes sight translation a very specific type of fast reading (taking in the text visually, focusing on some units and discerning only information which is useful). Sight translation is, for a translator according to some scholars (M. Brady 1989, W.K. Weber 1990) one of the most difficult and demanding types of translation. In some cases visual stimuli are complemented by auditory stimuli reaching the interpreter simultaneously, particularly in a growing number of situations where a speaker's address at a conference is complemented by a visual presentation to the audience, and where consecutive or simultaneous interpreting turns into sight translation. In these situations the highest degree of divisibility of attention is expected to be demonstrated by a translator. And, what is more, visual stimuli are so strong that it is in the sight translation where the interference reaches its highest level.

Sight translation is an interesting type of translation from a translation didactics, i.e. translodidactic point of view. For many years it has been applied to developing interpreting competences in both consecutive and simultaneous modes of interpreting. It can also be used to consolidate knowledge, to practise the translation reflex and the selection of translation techniques, etc… We should bear in mind, that at many European higher education institutions (including Germany) sight translation is a separate discipline on degree translation courses.

Referring to the experiment, it should be noted that the majority of students stated that they had not done translating or interpreting professionally before and over 50% of the subjects had not done any sight translating before (sight translation – neither classes nor lectures – does not figure in the Institute's course curriculum). However, many persons when asked about informal translating admitted to sight translating letters, emails, press texts or advertisements *ad hoc* for their family members or acquaintances.

5.

My previous paper (M. Płużyczka 2012a) drew on my pilot study results and included reflections on the possible scope of eye-tracking research in translation studies and ways of representing eye-tracking data. My current paper will briefly present concrete results of the research that has been carried out. I shall commence with a heat map that illustrates the duration of fixation for all subjects, in other words, the text elements on which the subjects fixated longest. These elements are marked in red:

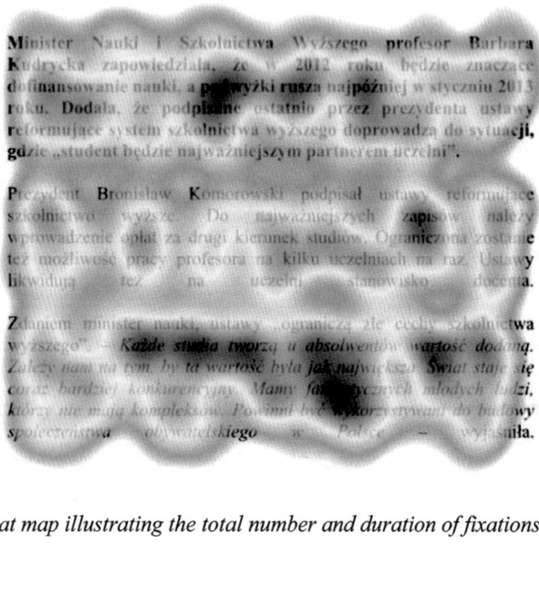

Fig.1. Heat map illustrating the total number and duration of fixations for all subjects

Duration of fixation, i.e. elements on which the subjects' eyes stopped longest, can also be illustrated on a gaze plot map. To demonstrate this I shall present a gaze plot map of the student who produced the highest number of fixations (the total number of fixations, including re-fixations, amounted in his case to 654):

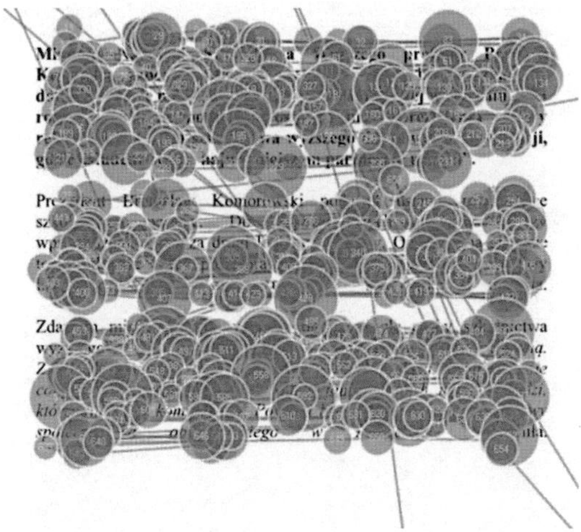

Fig.2. *A gaze plot map with the highest number of fixations and re-fixations*

In the case of a professional translator the total number of fixations amounted to 331:

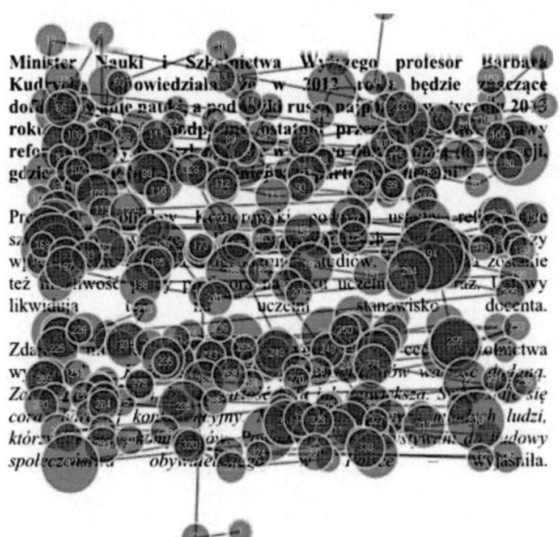

Fig.3. *A gaze plot map of the professional translator with a relatively low number of fixations registered in the experiment*

As presented (Fig. 2 and Fig. 3), the number of fixations registered by a professional translator was just half as much; and they were much shorter. (their duration is represented by the size of the diameter of a fixation circle).

The following map presents the longest fixations registered in this experiment:

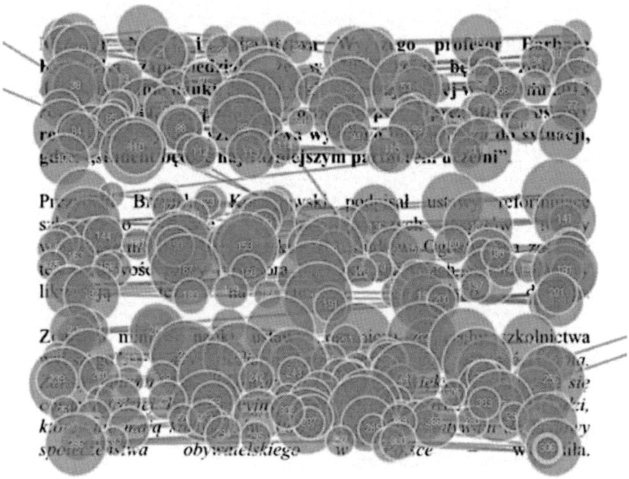

Fig.4. A gaze plot map of the student with the longest fixations

Interestingly enough, longer fixations did not result in a longer overall translation time. This resulted from a considerably lower number of fixations. In the case of this subject only 306 fixations were registered, which was the lowest number in the experiment. During the translation the subject (student) focused for a very long time on the words s/he was translating at a given moment, and did not return to previous words. Consequently, s/he had no re-fixations, which, in turn, slightly shortened the duration (3:08) of translation for the entire text, hence his/her time nearly equaled the average translation time for the experiment (the professional translator took 2:04 to translate the text).

For the purpose of comparison, I shall present one more gaze plot map, that of a student who registered the shortest fixations:

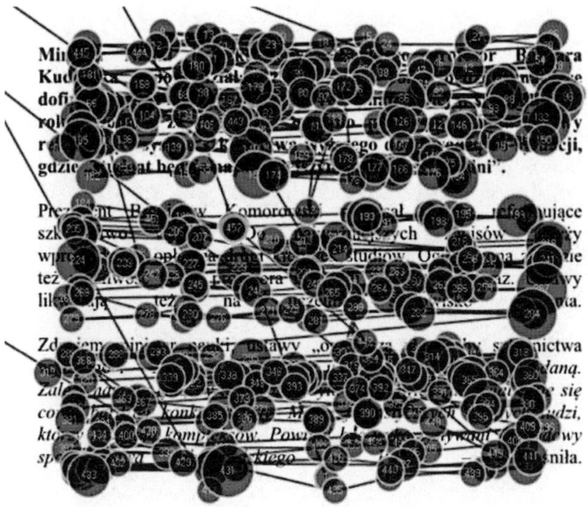

Fig.5. A gaze plot map of a subject with the shortest fixations

As presented, the number of fixations and re-fixations in this case was very high and amounted to 449, nevertheless the translation time was satisfactory – 2:35. The subject often moved his/her eyes sideways while attempting to retrieve from his/her memory a given word in Russian. This translation was however not satisfactory in terms of correctness.

As it turns out, the correctness of translation does not depend on the number and duration of fixations. It is the subject's manner of reading that determines these parameters; some subjects focus their eyes on the words that are being translated, some move them quickly over the words, and even beyond the text or screen. The two factors that determine a student's skill when dealing with a sight-translation task is the time spent on it and the level of correctness of the text delivered. Data analysis of the professionally delivered translation (P1-subject 1) supports this statement.

Regardless of the text reception manner, i.e. a lower or higher number of fixations, each subject focused longer on some text elements, and shorter on others. This gives rise to the question of why the subjects stopped their eyes on certain elements, and not on others. Since the source text was formulated in their mother tongue (A language), it seems highly unlikely, to the point of even being ruled out, that this resulted from reception problems. Generally speaking, longer fixations on certain words or larger text elements indicate that these elements constitute a translation difficulty. At least this is what the experiment showed.

6.

Let us now proceed and discuss the results of the first part of the analysis that was carried out. As graphically indicated on the above heat map the elements with the longest fixations, i.e. the elements which proved most difficult for students to render were:

- podwyżki ruszą najpóźniej w styczniu 2013 roku
- podpisane ostatnio przez prezydenta ustawy
- każde studia tworzą u absolwentów wartość dodaną
- zależy nam, by ta wartość była jak największa
- świat staje się
- mamy fantastycznych młodych ludzi

Let us analyze these text elements which received the longest fixations and ponder the reasons for this (for clarity of discussion fragments of the sentences presented above will be broken into smaller sentence elements).

1. *podwyżki*

In Polish the term *podwyżka* refers to a rise in salary; however, it is not enough to use its equivalent *повышение*, as the Russian word not only refers to an increase in monthly pay, but it may also refer an increase in quality, requirements, or something completely different. The expression that should be used in Russian is *повышение/увеличение/рост заработной платы* or *увеличение размера должностных окладов*. Therefore, a longer fixation resulted from a difficulty in translation stemming from unequal equivalent terms. However, in this text the term *podwyżka* can be classified as a specialized term. Consequently, the term *podwyżka* constitutes a difficulty in specialized term translation.

2. *podwyżki <u>ruszą</u>*

The word *ruszą* was one of the words which received the longest total fixation time for all the subjects. Due to the high speed at which information is received, processed, and then delivered in a foreign language, metaphors turn out to be the most serious translation problem for subjects (as proved by SMI eye tracker-supported research carried out by me in 2012). In the Polish text the word *ruszą* in the expression *podwyżki ruszą* was used with a metaphorical function. This metaphor cannot be expressed in Russian with the use of *увеличение заработной платы двинется* as this sentence fails to make any sense. Therefore, a longer fixation indicates that the students were considering either the use of another metaphor, or concretization of the concept expressed by *podwyżki ruszą* with the use of *повышение заработной платы произойдёт...*, thus abandoning the metaphor completely. Only a skillful and experienced translator is unlikely to have translation problems in such a situation, which, as a matter of fact, is what our eye-tracking research proved. Comparing the students' heat maps and that of the professional translator participating in the experiment, it should be noted that the translator's heat map did not show a longer fixation time on the element under discussion.

3. *najpóźniej*

Adverbs proved a serious translation difficulty in sight translation from Polish into Russian. This seems the perfect place to reflect on why. Is it linked to far too little attention being devoted to this part of speech in the process of translation didactics or, more generally, in the process of glottodidactics? A questionnaire-based survey, including a question referring to the teaching process, should provide an answer to this question.

In addition, *najpóźniej* is an adverb used in its superlative form, which may be indicative of a problem of a grammatical nature.

Translations of the sentence that included the discussed adverb contained content-related errors as well. The Polish sentence *...podwyżki ruszą najpóźniej w styczniu 2013 roku...* means that the pay rises will probably start earlier, but most definitely will have become fact by January 2013 (at the latest). One of the versions given was *не раньше чем* (literally *no earlier than*). This translation solution constitutes a content-related error, as it alters the meaning of the entire sentence. It can be assumed however, that in this case even a content-related error results from the students' inability to find an appropriate equivalent to this adverb, or from their insufficient skills in comparison of adverbs. The following cases of incorrect forms being used prove this assumption. Students, unable to grade adverbs correctly, produced in Russian grammatically incorrect forms: *в самом хужем случае, наипозже,* or even *наипозднее.*

4. *podpisane*

This is a past participle. Producing an appropriate form in Russian should not constitute a difficulty for Polish students. However, a longer fixation on this element, confirmed by a longer pause in audio-recording, can only be interpreted as a pause so as to think whether a shorter or longer form of a Russian participle should be used. This seems to be the case with the expression *ograniczona*. In both cases, despite a longer pause to think, the majority of students did not select the correct form. In the first case, when a participle is used to modify the noun – *podpisane przez prezydenta ostatnio ustawy* – a "longer" form of the participle (*подписанные*) should have been used in Russian. In the second case, in the phrase *ograniczona też zostanie możliwość pracy...* a short form of the participle (*ограничена*) should have been used, as it functions as a predicative in a complex predicate. Therefore, the above mistakes are of a grammatical (morphological) character. More attention should be drawn to them in translation teaching, as the short forms of adjectives (adjectival participles) do not seem natural to Poles. They are the remnants of the nominal declension of adjectives and occur very rarely in the Polish language. In Russian their usage depends on the word's function in a sentence, and very often on the meaning as well.

5. *podpisane przez*

The use of the expression *przez* in the phrase *podpisane przez* should be looked at from the syntactic point of view. The form *подписанные через президента, министра* does not conform to natural usage in Russian. The equivalent to the Polish construction *podpisane przez (kogoś)* is a participle and noun in the instrumental: *подписанные кем? – подписанные президентом, министром* determined categorically by a non-prepositional rection of the verb *подписать* (*кем?).*

6. *ostatnio*

This is yet another adverb that posed problems for the students. It should be pointed out that although this relatively long text contained just a few adverbs, students encountered problems with their rendition in all cases. This instance is particularly surprising, as the adverb *ostatnio* is a relatively frequently used word. Although it cannot be replaced with an exact single-word Russian equivalent, the expression *в последнее время* should be used. It must be emphasized that this is a very typical and commonly used Russian construction. In rendering this seemingly easy construction, an interferential error was also made one of the subjects used the word *остатнио*, a word non-existent in the Russian language.

7. *ustawy*

Here we have the case of a lack of knowledge of domain-specific terminology (although students had completed the 4th term of the undergraduate course in the language of politics and economics). Additionally, some of them also made errors of an interferential character. A vast number of students incorrectly used the word *уставы* ("false friend") as an equivalent to the Polish term *ustawy*, instead of using the correct word *законы*. This was one of the most frequently made interferential errors in the experiment.

8. *każde studia*

Difficulties in translation of the Polish phrase *każde studia* are of a more complex nature. With this expression achieving equivalence for the word *studia* constitutes the most difficult task. Very often an incorrect calque *студия* was used in Polish into Russian translation. The problem is due to the fact that there is no direct equivalent of the term *studia* in Russian. Communicative equivalence of the term *studia* can be delivered in Russian with the use of words *учёба, обучение*, or by applying the technique of generalization and making it more precise by adding *в университете – учёба в университете*. In certain contexts the technique of concretization can be applied and such words as *специальность, направление подготовки, факультет* etc., can be used. Still, it seems surprising that in the translodidactic or even glottodidactic process the students' attention was not drawn to such basic translation issues.

9. *tworzą u absolwentów*

What poses a problem in this case is finding a Russian equivalent to the verb *tworzą*, used in a metaphorical sense. Finding an equivalent to this element took students a long time, which only confirmed previous observations that students cannot apply translation techniques. The simplest translation solution to be implemented here was to replace the metaphor with a neutral expression *является*. Another problem in the analyzed phrase was the word *absolwent*, on which students stopped their eyes for a while. In most cases the subjects found a correct equivalent solution using the word *выпускник*, although that solution is not entirely correct, as in Russian the word *выпускник* requires an object: *выпускник чего? = выпускник вуза,* which means that arriving at an ideal translation solution would only require using an object, thus making it more precise. It should be added that the correctness of the use of *выпускник* on its own was context guaranteed, since it definitely referred to higher education institutions graduates. Only one person made an interferential error here by using the word *абсольвент*, which does not exist in the Russian language.

10. *wartość dodaną*

The sentence *Każde studia tworzą u absolwentów wartość dodaną* proved exceptionally difficult for students to translate. Its first part has already been analyzed above. Let us now take a closer look at the specialized term *wartość dodana*. It is obvious that this translation difficulty stems from the lack of knowledge of terminology in a foreign language. But that's not all. Using a term in a metaphoric meaning carries the risk that it may not be used metaphorically in the target language. Therefore, using another Russian expression that renders the concept seems to be the best solution. In this case students could say that every additional course of studies constitutes an additional asset or advantage: *Каждая следующая специальность является для выпускников вузов дополнительным преимуществом*. This case demonstrates that students have not assimilated translation techniques sufficiently, or at least the technique of paraphrasing (which involves restating the meaning using other words when the direct equivalent is not known. This, after all, constitutes the basis of translation competence. This seems the right place to stop and reflect on whether there exist some gaps in the translodidactic system, and whether specially prepared exercises should be introduced in the first few years of the translation course to develop such skills in future students adept in the art of translation.

11. *mamy fantastycznych młodych ludzi*

Hesitation (evidenced with longer fixations and pauses in the audio-recording) while translating this sentence could have resulted from the fact that when the word *fantastic* "entered" the Russian language, it was initially used to mean fantasy or science fiction. Students were probably afraid of making an interferential error since they were uncertain whether they were using a calque or whether the word *фантастический* had started to be used in Russian with the meaning "splendid, wonderful, outstanding, great"[9]. Indeed, the option *фантастические* meaning "great" is closer to colloquial language and therefore the options: *замечательные, талантливые, перспективные, многообещающие* would definitely be better and more correct in this case.

12. *doprowadzą do*

This expression, as one of the very few in the text received one of the longest fixations. It was quite unexpected for me that such a variety of errors were made in its rendering: a grammatical error (incorrect conjugation), a lexical error (a lack of knowledge of the equivalent and the use of an incorrect expression), an interferential error (*допроважут*), and a syntactic error (application of incorrect verb rection: *доведут к..., приведут до....*) all occurred.

13. *w styczniu 2013*

Numerals and their declension have always posed problems for translators. As in the cases above, a question arises: should even more attention be given to this issue? Particularly, as numerals seem to constitute a translation problem in any foreign language. Russian is not an exception to this rule; on the contrary, I dare say, it is numerals' declension that is among the most difficult in any language.

14. *zapisy*

In this case the translation problem pertained to inadequate knowledge of specialized terminology, although that was not the only problem. The rendition of the term *zapisy* exposed students' inability to approach a translation task in a situation, where they are not familiar with an equivalent of a particular

9 *ФАНТАСТИ́ЧЕСКИЙ, -ая, -ое.: **1.** см.* фантастика. ***2.** Похожий на фантазию* (*во 2* знач.); *причудливый, волшебный, сверхъестественный.* Ф. пейзаж. Фантастическое освещение. ***3.** Совершенно неправдоподобный, невероятный, несбыточный.* Фантастическая новость. Фантастически (нареч.) умён кто-н. ***4.*** Исключительный (*в 3* знач.), удивительный (*во 2* знач.) (разг.). Ф. нахал. (http://www.ozhegov.org/words/37978.shtml).

expression, in other words, their inability to apply translation techniques. As in the case of the term *wartość dodana*, a longer fixation failed to result in an appropriate translation solution. Nearly all the students used the word *записы*, a word that does not exist in Russian, thus making an error of an interferential character. The following translation solutions can apply here: the word *zapisy* can be replaced with the equivalent *положения* or, alternatively, a process of either concretization or generalization via *нормы, принципы, правила,* or *принципы установления/введения оплат* can be applied, as the fragment referred to a bill introducing tuition fees for students doing a second university degree course.

The "problem areas" described above and graphically presented on the heatmaps and gaze plots, allowed us to reveal subjects' (students') sight translation difficulties. The analysis also highlights areas of language competence and translation-related knowledge that should be given particular attention in the translodidactic process.

The first stage of the lapsological analysis of the experiment's results involved a selection of text fragments on which the subjects fixated longest, i.e. those posing difficulties for them, and an explanation of translation-related difficulties created by theses fragments. The second stage involved the compilation and categorization of their errors based on the audio recordings of the subjects, which will be addressed below. Not only did this identify the main areas of difficulty for the subjects; it enabled us to characterise sight translation in lapsological terms.

In the section below, I shall introduce the error analysis results and categorize the errors made by the subjects.

7.

Eye-tracking-aided experiments allow researchers to video-record movements of the subjects' eye balls and to make audio recordings of the orally rendered text. Comparing these two types of recordings enables us to compile and categorize subjects' translation errors. The resulting data analysis (of 17 translated texts) confirmed a previously formulated hypothesis that interferential errors constitute a large percentage of errors made in sight translation. Even so, their number exceeded initial expectations.

Chart 1: *interferential errors*

Polish expression	Incorrect equivalent	Number of errors[10]	Correct Russian equivalent
1. ustawa	устав	13 (5)	закон
2. minister	министер	9 (8)	министр
3. studia	студия	7 (5)	обучение в университете, учёба в университете, специальность, направление подготовки
4. fantastyczni młodzi ludzie	– фантастические молодые люди – фантастичные люди	9 2	замечательные/талантливые/перспективные/многообещающие молодые люди
5. zapisy (w ustawie)	записы	8	положения, нормы, принцы, правила, принципы установления/введения оплат
6. ograniczona zostanie…	огран**ичают**...	5	ограничивают
7. na uczelni wyższej	**на** вузе	4	в вузе
8. na uniwersytecie	**на** университете	3	в университете
9. absolwent	абсольвент	3	выпускник вуза
10. zależy nam na	нам зависит на	3	для нас важным является
11. podwyżka	– повышение – подвысшение зарплат	2 1	повышение/увеличение заработной платы, увеличение размера должностных окладов, рост заработной платы
12. zdaniem minister	– по мнению минист**ер** – по мнению мини**стр**	2 1	по мнению министра
13. konkurencyjny	– конкуренцийный – конкуренционный – конкурентивный	1 1 1	конкурентный
14. wykorzystani	использован**и**	2	использованы
15. świat staje się	– мир стается – мир стает	1 1	становится

10 The numbers in brackets refer to the number of subjects who made a given error. This numbers differ from the number of errors, as certain words occur more than once in the text.

16. minister nauki i szkolnictwa wyższego	– Министер **эдукации** и высшего образования – Министер науки и высшего образования	1 1	министр науки и высшего образования
17. dofinansowanie	дофинансование	1	дополнительное финансирование, дофинансирование
18. najpóźniej	найпозже	1	позже всего
19. doprowadzą	допроважут	1	приведут к...
20. wprowadzenie (opłat)	впровождение	1	введение, установление (оплаты)
21. ostatnio	остатнио	1	в последнее время
22. system	систем	1	система
23. drugi kierunek	**другое** направление	1	второй факультет
24. szkolnictwo wyższe	высшая эдукация	1	высшее образование
25. (…) możliwość pracy profesora…	возможность **працы** профессора	1	возможность **работы** профессора
26. stanowisko docenta	**становиско** доцента	1	должность доцента
27. możliwości	можливости	1	возможности
28. do najważniejszych zapisów …	к **найважнейшим** записам ...	1	к самым важным положениям самые важные положения
29. złe cechy	вады	1	плохие черты
30. podpisane przez prezydenta	подписанные **через** президента	1	подписанные президентом
31. młodzi ludzie	млодые люди	1	молодые люди
32. wartość	**вартость**	1	ценность
33. społeczeństwa obywatelskiego	**обывательского** общества	1	гражданского общества
34. była jak największa	была **как** найбольшей	1	была самой большой
35. podpisał ustawy	была подписана закон	1	был подписан закон

The above examples prove that in some cases interferential errors are at times surprising as they occur in seemingly easy translation cases. However, this is the risk of sight translating – having so little time or being under time pressure, and being affected by such a strong stimulus as the visual stimulus is, translators are highly influenced by the written text. As the results of the experiment show, interferential errors are the errors which are made most frequently in sight translation If these results were to be compared with the two modes of interpreting (consecutive and simultaneous) in terms of frequency of interferential error occurrence, then, based on my own experience in teaching both translating and interpreting, I would state that interferential errors definitely occur less frequently in the case of interpreting. This may be attributed to the fact that that both reception and production are realized by means of the same channel, i.e. an auditory-verbal channel, whereas in the case of sight translation the difficulty of simultaneity lies in the fact that these channels are different – the source language text is in a written form, whereas the target language text is concurrently produced orally. Drawing a comparison between the results of this experiment with those of the experiment investigating errors in written translation, carried out by me in 2008 (M. Płużyczka 2009, 2011), it should be stated that, by contrast, interferential errors are relatively rare in written translation.

When faced with such a high number of interferential errors one feels induced to arrive at conclusions of a translodidactic nature. Sadly enough, it should be stated that the students often made these errors because of their highly deficient knowledge of appropriate vocabulary, including specialised vocabulary, and instead of using one of the translation techniques applicable in such cases (e.g. descriptive equivalent, antonymic translation, etc.), they produced calques and used polonisms. Neither of the latter applications belongs to translation techniques to be used by translators when they do not know the direct equivalent in a foreign language, or when they are faced with non-equivalent lexis. As exemplified, it is evident that students do not know translation techniques, they are not taught about them and trained to use them, and when not familiar with the equivalent, they cannot find and apply a correct translation solution.

What's more, a comparison with heat maps and gaze plots revealed that quite frequently the subjects failed to register longer fixations at the moment of making interferential errors, which indicates that they were not aware they were making such errors. This implies they do not have a habit acquired by means of practising translation, even doing sight translation, and they have not yet developed a reflex that could prevent them from making such errors.

Another interesting case identified in the experiment is indirect interference, i.e. being influenced not by the word which occurs in the Polish text, but by its synonym which exists in the source language, e.g. the term *министр эдукации* was used to render the expression *minister nauki*, or *вады* to render *złe cechy* included in the Polish text. Errors of this type also include calques of word combinations prepositional phrases etc., e.g. ***на*** *вузе,* ***на*** *университете,* or errors in conjugation resulting from the influence of the Polish language, e.g. *ограничивают* etc.

To sum up, the number of interferential errors amounted to 100 out of the total number of 203 errors made in the experiment. This means that interferential errors constitute nearly half of all errors that occured in the translation.

To sum up, the number of interferential errors amounted to 100 out of the total number of 203 errors made in the experiment. This means that interferential errors constitute nearly half of all errors that occured in the translation.

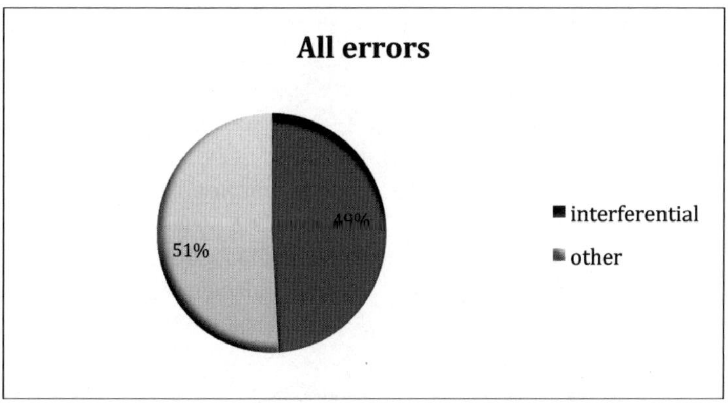

All errors	203		
Interferential errors	100	lexical	78
		grammatical	22
Other	103		

Lexical interferential errors accounted for 78 percent of all interferential errors, while the share of grammatical interferential errors amounted to 22 percent.

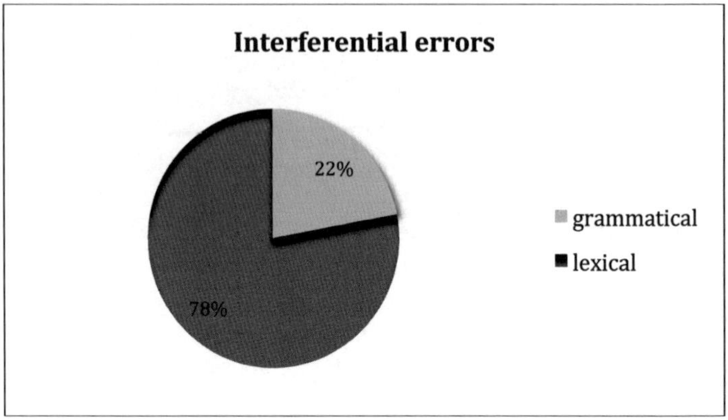

Grammatical errors constituted the second type of errors analysed in the experiment carried out. Some of these errors were quite unanticipated, but at the same time interesting since they show which language areas pose a difficulty to the subjects. These are among others: adjective and adverb comparison and also word collocation, verb agreement, and even conjugation and declension. Some cases are classified as both grammatical and interferential errors.

Chart 2: grammatical errors

Section of the text in Polish	Section of the translated text including the error	Number of errors	Correct version	Type of error
1. była jak największa	– была как найбольшей – была как возможно найболее – была **как** лучше – была как больше – была как можно большая – была все большая	1 1 1 1 1 1	была самой большой	error in adjective grading
2. ograniczona zostanie…	огран**ичают**...	5	ограничивают	error in verb conjugation
3. zależy nam na	– нам зависит на том – мы хо**чем**	3 1	– для нас важным является то – мы хотим	lexical error, language calque, error in conjugation

4. na uczelni wyższej	на вузе	4	в вузе	incorrect choice of a preposition; interferential error
5. na uniwersytecie	на университете	3	в университете	incorrect choice of a preposition; interferential error
6. doprowadzą do (sytuacji)	– доведет **к** – вызов**ит** ситуацию – (приведут) к ситуац**ию**	3 1 1	приведут к ситуаци, доведут до ситуации	– error in collocation – error in conjugation – declensional error
7. zdaniem minister	– по мнению минист**ер** – по мнению мини**стр**[11]	2 1	по мнению министра	declensional error, interferential error: feminine declension instead of masculine
8. wykorzystani	использован**и**	2	использованы	interferential error, Polish ending in the participle
9. zdaniem minister	по министру	2	по словам министра	syntactic error
10. najpóźniej	– позднее – найпозже	1 1	позже всего	error in adverb grading
11. świat staje się	– мир стается – мир стает	1 1	мир становится	error in verb conjugation
12. system	систем	1	система	masculine gender instead of feminine; interferential error
13. na kilku uczelniach	на больше одного вуза	1	на нескольких вузах	incorrect declension of a comparable adverbial structure;also a lexical error as a direct target language equivalent to a neumeral pronoun could have been found
14. do najważniej-szych	в ряд**е** самых важных	1	в ряду	declensional error
15. wprowadzenie opłat	внедрение оплачиван**ие**	1	введение оплат	lexical and declensional error

11 Interference consisting in appying a feminine form to the word министр, which in Russian exists only as a masculine noun.

16.	ograniczą złe cechy	уменьш**ится** плохие черты	1	ограничат/ уменьшат плохие свойства	conjugational error
17.	złe cechy	плохое черты	1	плохие черты	incorrect ending of an adjective; not suitable for a noun in the plural
18.	podpisał ustawy	был**а** подписан**а** закон	1	был подписан закон	error in noun gender, interferential error
19.	ustawy likwidują	закон будут ликвидировать	1	законы будут ликвидировать	noun and verb disagreement in number
20.	powinni być wykorzysty-wani do budowy	должны быть использованы в строе**ние**	1	для создания	declensional error
21.	podpisane przez prezydenta	подписанные **через** президента	1	подписанные президентом	incorrect case government
22.	ustawy	закона	1	законы	incorrect consruction of plural form

As in the case of simultaneous interpreting, grammatical errors are made frequently during sight translation. Both types of rendition are performed very fast, with little time to think over the correctness of the form applied. However, this does not mean these are the "standard" situations. That is why a well-trained translator should be equipped with well internalized (deeply rooted) grammatical structures so that appropriate grammatical patterns "occur" automatically, so to speak, with no conscious morphological and syntactic analysis. What this means from a translodidactic point of view is that the process of teaching translators cannot be devoid of specialist training regarding their grammatical competences and that the so-called (neo)communicative approach, so widely promoted, does in this particular respect more harm than good. To sum up the above reflections, one should state that a well-trained interpreter and sight translator should be able to produce a target language text that is also grammatically correct. In short, what makes a sight translator/interpreter a good sight translator/interpreter is his/her ability to produce a text that is also grammatically correct. The fact that sight translation may, due to its very nature, bring about grammatical and/or interferential errors is a separate issue.

When analysing the percentage share of grammatical errors made during sight translation one should arrive at the conclusion that this type of errors does not occur as frequently as lexical errors or terminological errors, which are made most frequently.

All errors	203		
Lexical	154	Terminological	106
		Other	48
Grammatical	49		

Lexical errors constitute as much as 76 percent of all errors. Grammatical errors constitute the remaining 24 percent.

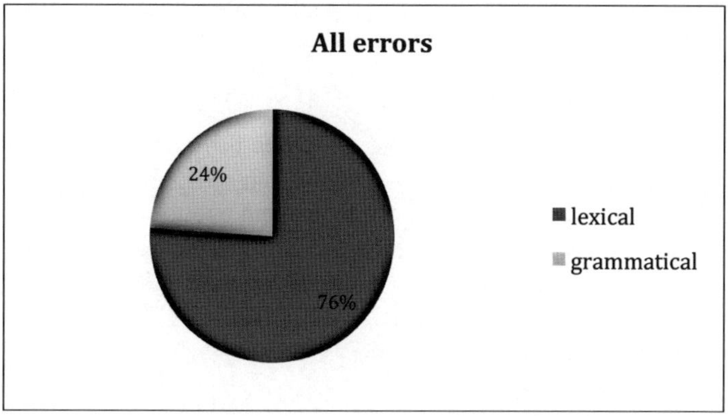

When it comes to lexical errors, terminological errors constitute the overwhelming majority (69 percent).

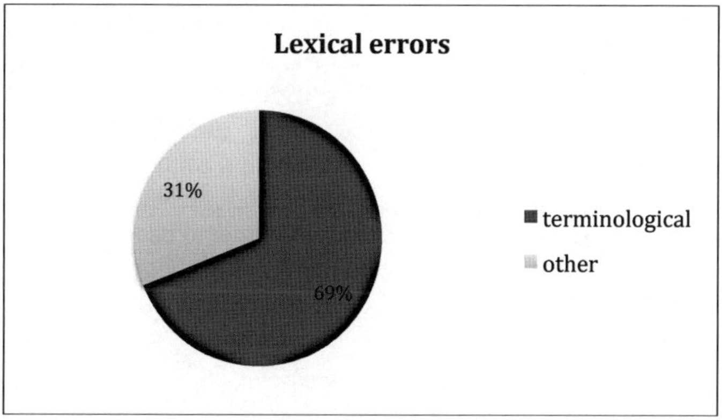

Errors relating to the use of specialized vocabulary, or terminological errors, constituted the third group of errors, specified below:

Chart 3: terminological errors

Section of the text in Polish	Section of the translated text including the error	Number of errors	Correct version
1. ustawa	– устав – указ – договор	13 (5) 3 (1) 3 (1)	закон
2. szkolnictwo wyższe	– высшее обучение – высшее учебные заведения – высшая эдукация – обучение	5 (3) 3 (2) 3 (1) 1	высшее образование
3. podwyżka	– brak ekwiwalentu – повышение – подвысшение – большая оплата – большая зарплата для работников – подвысшение зарплат – повышение фондов – взвышки зарплат – субсидия – больше денег	5 2 1 1 1 1 1 1 1 1	повышение/увеличение заработной платы, увеличение размера должностных окладов, рост заработной платы
4. studia	– студия – курсы – образование	7 (5) 2 1	обучение в университете, учёба в университете, специальность, направление подготовки
5. stanowisko (docenta)	– пост доцента – становиско доцента – работа доцента – звание доцента – степень доцента – возможность работать доктором – доценцкая аспирантура	6 2 2 1 1 1 1	должность доцента
6. zapisy (w ustawie)	– записы – указы – уставы – правила	8 1 1 1	положения, нормы, принципы, правила, принципы установления/ введения оплат ... (zapisy wprowadzające opłaty za drugi kierunek)

7. konkurencyjny (świat)	– конкурентноспособный – конкурентивный – конкуренционный – конкуренцийный	3 1 1 1	мир становится более конкурентным
8. obywatelskie (społeczeństwo)	– (opuszczenie/ pominięcie) – обывательское	5 1	гражданское общество
9. nauka	просвещение учеба освещение	1 1 1	наука
10. absolwent	абсольвент	3	выпускник вуза
11. uczelnia	школа заведение	1 1	вуз
12. kierunek	курс	2	факультет, направление подготовки, специальность

Again, this was a surprising result. The terms used in the source text were neither complicated nor little known. As mentioned previously, the text was selected so that the specialized vocabulary it included should be commonly known to persons familiar with the life of the areas where the target language is spoken.

The subjects also made many (purely) lexical errors. They were as follows:

Chart 4: lexical errors

Polish phrase or word	**Section of the translated text including the error**	**Number of errors**	**Correct version**
1. nam zależy	нам зависит на том	3	для нас очень важным является ...
2. fantastycznych ludzi	– фантастические люди – фантастичные люди – благоприятные	9 2 1	замечательные/талантливые/перспективные/многообещающие молодые люди
3. dofinansowanie	– дофинансование – дофинансировка – финансировки	1 1 2	дополнительное финансирование, дофинансирование
4. doprowadzą	– допроваджут – довести к ситуации – довезёт (до ситуации)	1 1 1	приведут к...
5. zdaniem minister	по министру	2	по словам министра

6. wprowadzenie (opłaty)	– впровождение – внедрение	1 1	введение, установление (оплаты)
7. świat staje się	– мир стается – стает	1 1	становится
8. ostatnio	остатнио	1	в последнее время
9. opłata za (drugi kierunek)	введение **зарплаты** за	1	введение оплаты за ...
10. drugi kierunek	**другое** направление	1	второй факультет
11. (…) możliwość pracy profesora…	возможность **працы** профессора	1	возможность работы профессора/занятности профессора
12. możliwości	можливости	1	возможности
13. złe cechy	вады	1	плохие черты
14. wartość	вартость	1	ценность
15. budowa (społeczeństwa)	– стройка общества – троение	1 1	создание общества

However, I would like to draw particular attention to an error in the translation/transposition of proper names, in this case to the name of a performed political function. I was deeply astonished to “see” so many incorrect renditions of this name. Bearing in mind that classes in the language of politics figure in the curriculum of the first and second year of the course, students should have been familiar with this function and its name.

16. Minister Nauki i Szkolnictwa Wyższego	– Минист**ер** **образования** и высшего **обучения** – Министр науки и **вузов** – Министр высшего образования – Минист**ер** **эдукации** и высшего образования – Министр **учебы** и высшего **обучения** – Министер **учебы** и высшего образования – Минист**ер** науки и высшего	2 1 1 1 1 1 1	Министр науки и высшего образования

	образования – Министр образования – Министер освещения – Министр обучения	 3 1 1	

The final group is made up of content-related errors – translation errors which are considered the most serious. In the case of sight translation it is commonly believed (M. Brady 1989, D. Gile 2009, W.K. Weber 1990) that since the translated text is constantly in front of the translator, the information expressed by it, or its sections, is constantly "available,, to the translator (on the monitor) and, as a consequence, the translator does not make (or should not make), or makes only minor, content-related errors. In the chart below, the subjects' content-related errors are listed. The experiment and the resulting data analysis do not fully support the above mentioned view. That said, why, despite the constant availability of information, does a sight translator still make content-related errors?

Chart 5: content-related errors

Section of the text in Polish	**Incorrect version of translation in Russian**
Ustawy likwidują też na uczelni stanowisko docenta.	**Уставы** ликвидируют **работу** доцента в вузе. (2) Законы ликвидируют тоже **аспирантуру.** Законы ликвидируют тоже **докторскую аспирантуру.** **Устав** ликвидирует также **звание доцента** в вузе. Законы ликвидируют тоже **возможность работать доктором** в университете. Эти законы ликвидируют тоже **степень доцента** в вузах.
(...) a podwyżki ruszą najpóźniej w styczniu 2013 roku.	(…) **большая зарплата** для работников будет **не раньше** чем в январе 2013 г.
Każde studia tworzą u absolwentów wartość dodaną.	Каждые студия **сделают** для выпцускников **добавочную стоимость.**
Dodała, że podpisane ostatnio przez prezydenta ustawy reformujące system szkolnictwa wyższego doprowadzą do sytuacji, gdzie „student będzie najważniejszym partnerem	Уставы **будут иметь результат в ситуации когда** студент будет самым важным партнером вуза.

uczelni".	
Ograniczona zostanie też możliwość pracy profesora na kilku uczelniach na raz.	Ограниченная будет тоже работа профессора в нескольких вузах **на один раз.**
Zależy nam na tym, by ta wartość była jak największa.	**Нам зависит на том, чтобы** эта **стоимость** была как **можно большею**.
Powinni być wykorzystywani do budowy społeczeństwa obywatelskiego w Polsce.	Молодые люди в Польше **должны работать над нашей страной.**

It is my opinion that the analysis of errors made by the subjects allows us to claim that content-related errors resulted to a large extent from the subjects' insufficient language competence as the subjects did not know how to deal with a particular language situation, and which equivalent to apply; they attempted to construct a sentence in a different way, often losing the meaning of the utterance at the same time. Still, another research experiment is required to prove this claim.

8.

The above charts show the errors most commonly made by students in the process of sight translation, the encountered areas of difficulty, and, most importantly, their attempts at dealing with such a difficulty; i.e. whether they are approaching it correctly, and whether they are losing the meaning of the utterance at the same time. The analysis shows that students make numerous lexical and grammatical errors, which result from their insufficient language competence. One should reflect here on how to make the translodidactic process more efficient, focusing more on the problem areas.

Language interference proved to be a serious translation-related problem. Not only did the subjects succumb to lexical interference but quite often they were transferring grammatical structures typical of the Polish language into Russian and using the formed constructions in Russian. The following are the two main issues that require attention here: firstly, the words that often undergo interference and, secondly, the ways of approaching and dealing with elements with no target language equivalents. The fact that so many subjects used polonisms may be attributed to their conviction that it may be the simplest method of dealing with a troublesome translation situation. Needless to say, such reasoning is wrong and may lead to incorrect habits.

The experiment also shows how poorly students perform while doing sight translation, a seemingly easy type of translation. What can be inferred from this is the fact that instruction in sight translation should be introduced to translation didactics on a systematic basis and with the application of a separate curriculum. It should be added that exercises in sight translation also develop translators' reflexes. Moreover, this type of translation allows for time-effective and relatively easy verification of students' particular skills and competences.

To conclude: owing to the fact that eye-tracking research into sight translation (in this case the translation of a Polish text into Russian) shows the elements on which the subjects (in this case students) stop their eyes longest, it can be determined what kind of information is most difficult for the subjects to process; in other words, what poses (the most serious) translation difficulties for them. Moreover, eye-tracking recording reveals their skills but also, and probably most importantly, their inability to deal with certain translation situations.

Arriving at applicative conclusions in the form of a relevant *translodidactic curriculum* shall be a subsequent stage of a comprehensive and systematic eye-tracking analysis of sight translation.

References

Brady, M. (1989): *Case studies in sight translation.* In: J. Dodds (ed.), The Theoretical and Practical Aspects of Teaching Conference Interpretation. Udine. 141–243.

Göpferich, S./ Jääskeläinen, R. (2009): *Process research into the development of translation competence: Where are we, and where do we need to go?* In: S. Göpferich/ R. Jääskeläinen (eds), Process Research into Translation Competence. Special Issue of Across Languages and Cultures. 10 (2). 169–191.

Gile, D. (2009/ 1995): Basic Concepts and Models for Interpreter and Translator Training, Amsterdam/ Philadelphia.

Grucza, S. (2011): *Lingwistyka antropocentryczna a badania okulograficzne*. In: Lingwistyka Stosowana/ Applied Linguistics / Angewandte Linguistik. 4. 147–162.

Grucza, S. (2012): *The Investigation of Translation Competences and Translation Processes.* In: Vestnik MGLU, Moscow (in press).

Płużyczka, M. (2009a), *Psycholingwistyczne aspekty dydaktyki translacji tekstów specjalistycznych (na materiale rosyjskich tekstów prawnych)*. University of Warsaw. Warszawa (unpublished PhD Thesis).

Płużyczka, M. (2009b): *Dydaktyka translacji tekstów specjalistycznych – aspekt metodyczny.* In: Publikacja jubileuszowa II. W kręgu problematyki technolektalnej, Warszawa. 285–312.

Płużyczka, M. (2009c): *Dydaktyka translacji – rozważania terminologiczne.* In: Przegląd Glottodydaktyczny. 26. 195–200.

Płużyczka, M. (2011a): *Eye–Tracking–Analysen in der Translationswissenschaft. Zum Stand der Forschung*. In: Kwartalnik Neofilologiczny. LVIII. 4/ 2011. 473–484.

Płużyczka, M. (2011b): *Okulograficzne wsparcie badań nad procesem tłumaczenia a vista.* In: Lingwistyka Stosowana/ Applied Linguistics/ Angewandte Linguistik. 4. 180–189.

Płużyczka, M. (2011c): *Wybrane trudności translacyjne a proces translodydaktyczny*. In: O nauczaniu i uczeniu się języka dla potrzeb zawodowych. Lublin. 88–97.

Płużyczka, M. (2012a): *Eye–tracking Support of Translation Processes Analysis*. In: Vestnik MGLU, Moscow (in press).

Płużyczka, M. (2012b): *Na co patrzy, a co widzi tłumacz a vista? Translatoryczne możliwości poznawcze okulografii*. In: Lingwistyka Stosowana/ Applied Linguistics/ Angewandte Linguistik. 5. 65–74.

Weber, W. K. (1990): *The Importance of Sight Translation in an Interpreter Training Program*. In: American Translators Association Scholarly Monograph Series 4. Interpreting – Yesterday, Today and Tomorrow, D. & M. Bowen (eds). State University of New York. Binghamton N.Y. 44–52.

Internet sources

http://www.rosbalt.ru/moscow/2011/03/28/833118.html

http://dobrebadania.pl/slownik-badawczy.html?s=1

http://tvp.info/informacje/polska/podwyzki-dla-naukowcow-za-dwa-lata/4275578

http://gams.uni-graz.at/fedora/get/container:tc/bdef:Container/get

http://eyetracking.pl/

http://www.ozhegov.org/words/37978.shtml

Proactive Use of Eye-Tracking in the Translational Workflow

Silvia Hansen-Schirra (University Mainz/Germersheim)
Christoph Rösener (Flensburg University of Applied Sciences)

1. Introduction

For many years eye tracking has been used mainly for research purposes. In psychological research eye-tracking provided the data basis for testing empirically human perceptual or cognitive processes. At the same time eye-tracking was applied to marketing research for testing software usability or the effectiveness of marketing materials. Additionally, it was also used to study the handling of graphical user interfaces. All these approaches analyse data which was recorded before by the eye tracker. To use eye-tracking as a possibility to control or operate an application in real-time is a relatively new development. In the past very few applications, which were based on real gaze-assistance, were designed most of the time only for disabled people to give them control on functions of proprietary software (e. g. selecting objects, control menus, writing).

The use of gaze-assistance in conventional software programs – especially in the area of translational aids – is very new. One of the very interesting approaches towards conventional applications, which use gaze-assistance, is the iDict System (cf. A. Hyrskykari et al. 2000, 2003]. iDict is a translation aid for reading documents written in a foreign language. iDict observes the reader's eye movements and behaves proactively by providing help when the user has comprehension problems. The problems are identified by fixation duration and regression during the reading process. As soon as the user hesitates while reading a word or a phrase the embedded dictionaries are automatically consulted and a gloss and a dictionary entry, in the text or in a separate dictionary frame respectively, are displayed. The idea of iDict – to give aid in the moment the users' eye-gaze shows some comprehension problems – has also been tested in the Eye-to-IT project (cf. A. L. Jakobsen 2009), which is in turn very similar to the approaches we describe in the present paper. The methods used in iDict form the basis of our investigations of proactive use of eye-tracking in the translational workflow.

In this paper we will describe some new ideas for the use of gaze-assisted interaction in modern translational workflow. Starting from software applications which are used in the translational workflow we will distinguish three stages of the general process: before, during and after translation. Apart from potential locations for gaze-assisted interaction in the process we will present some proposals for the software design of translational aids as well as for suitable types of interactivity. After that we will give an interpretation of some eye-tracking data recorded in a session with translational software during the actual translation process. Furthermore, we will present the results of a case study, which shows possible fields of gaze-assisted interaction in connection with corpus linguistics. Finally, we will show how eye-tracking can be used in order to evaluate and improve the post-editing of machine translation.

2. Modern translational workflow

The modern translational workflow is dominated by the use of computers and software respectively. So called language technology tools are used in almost every single step of the translational process – from the initial creation of a text to the delivery of the final translation. Already during the creation of a text – before the actual translation – several language technology tools are used. First of all the text processing program itself. Multilingual text processing systems allow the handling of text in different languages providing different character sets and directions of writing. Moreover, most of these systems provide inbuilt spell and grammar checking as well as special plug-ins for dictionary, thesaurus or terminology database look-up. Additionally, especially in the area of technical documentation, authoring tools, also known as 'Controlled Language Tools', are used as aids for the creation of texts. Combined with linguistic intelligence besides spell and grammar checking, authoring tools are used to check abbreviations, style and terminology in texts. In most cases this is done in relation to special style guides – e.g. Simplified English, technical writing rules etc. – and terminology, most of the time both designated by the respective customer. Moreover linguistically intelligent authoring aids also can help the author to extract so called term candidates.

The translational process itself then is dominated by the use of translation memory systems. The results of various surveys indicate clearly that nowadays the majority of translators and translation companies, respectively, use translation memory systems during translation (cf. E. Lagoudaki 2006, A. Lommel 2004). Translation memory systems store whole sentences or clauses (called segments) and their translations in a translation memory. When the translator is translating a new document the segments are matched against those already present in the translation memory and the translator can reuse the matches found immediately for his new translation. At the same time most of the translation memory systems provide also a separate inbuilt terminology database. With the help of this database terminology can be managed and used for a parallel look-up during the matching process of the translation memory system.

For translation tasks which are highly repetitive and conventionalized or for internal communication purposes, machine translation is nowadays also implemented as preparatory translation step (cf. T. Gassmann 2009). The output is then post-edited by translators. Within this context, eye-tracking and key logging are used as evaluation tools for the machine translation output (cf. S. Doherty et al. 2010). Moreover, the productivity of post-editing processes can be predicted with these methods (cf. S. O'Brien 2011). They help to pave the way for the development of efficient human-aided machine translation systems.

So the use of language technology tools in modern translational workflow is manifold, thus providing many possibilities for gaze-assisted interaction. To describe the possible implementations of gaze-assisted interaction into modern translational workflow in the following it is necessary to distinguish three stages of the process: before, during and after translation.

3. Use of gaze-assisted interaction before translation

Text processing systems together with their inbuilt language technology functions are interesting in relation to gaze-assisted interaction. Especially the plug-in functions for dictionary, thesaurus or terminology database look-up could be done using gaze assistance. This approach is already described in detail by A. Hyrskykari (cf. A. Hyrskykari et. al. 2000, 2003). Therefore the present paper focuses on the possible use of gaze-assistance with authoring tools, also known as 'Controlled Language Tools', which, especially in the area of technical documentation, are used to write technical documents in relation to style guides and given terminology. With the help of software like, for example, the CLAT system the author – after writing a passage of text – can perform several quality checks (spelling, grammar, style and terminology) of the document (cf. IAI 2009a, 2009b). The problems found by the software are then marked in the text and on demand a special error message window (CLAT Navigator) is shown with further information (cf. Fig. 1).

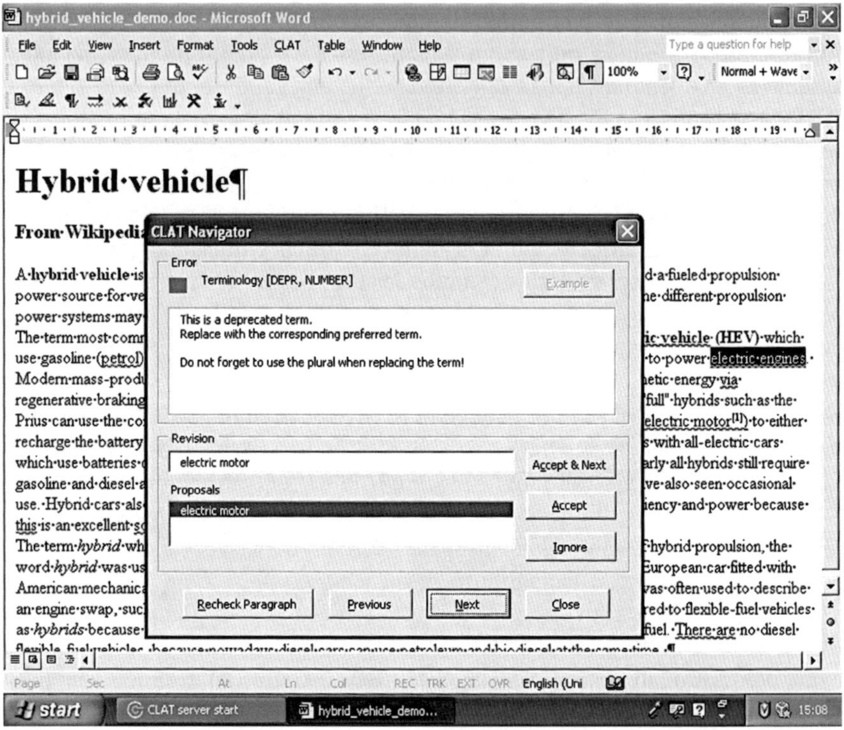

Fig. 1.: *CLAT Navigator window [Rösener 2010]*

Some of the mistakes the program marks might not be of interest to the author due to special circumstances in which the text is published or due to special language or style used in the written text. But the function "Next" provided by the software only allows one to jump from one error in the text to the next. To look up certain errors and activate the corresponding error message window individually is not very comfortable to handle.

Fulfilling this requirement using gaze-assistance would be a significant improvement of the user friendliness of the software. The software identifies problems in the text passage and marks them with a special colour code distinguished by the type of error. The idea is then that the author can trigger the CLAT Navigator window corresponding to the error of interest simply by using gaze-assistance. When the eye-tracker identifies a long fixation of a marked passage in the text by the user and the fixation exceeds a defined threshold limit, then the CLAT Navigator window which corresponds to the appropriate error, is shown. Unfortunately, at this time of the project, we cannot present proper research results for this application scenario, because the investigations concerning the use of gaze-assistance together with authoring tools are still under way at Mainz University.

4. Use of gaze assisted interaction during translation

Although the translational process is dominated by the use of translation memory systems, from the eye-tracking point of view it is worthwhile to take a short look at the terminology workflow as well.

4.1 Bilingual terminology/word clouds

In translation projects a terminology database is often provided by the customer. Occasionally this database consists of bilingual terminology. This is another possibility of using gaze-assistance in modern translational workflow. Using the above mentioned method of identifying long fixations bilingual terminology information can also be requested by the user simply by looking at the appropriate term. The bilingual term information is then displayed in an extra pop-up window. Additionally, further information can be given in the target language by not only displaying the corresponding term but entire word clouds, thus introducing the translator to the semantic field of the given term in the specific target language (cf. Fig. 2). Again, this application scenario is currently in its research phase and therefore proper results are not available yet.

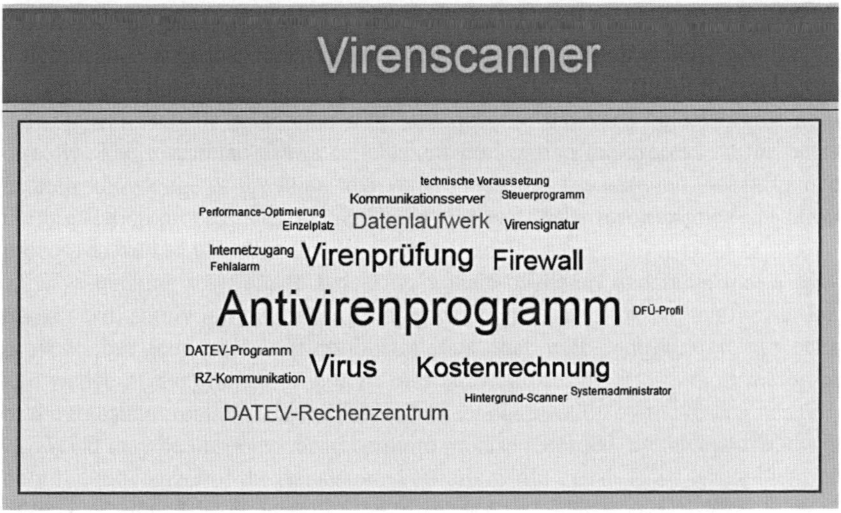

Fig. 2: Word cloud example for the German word "Virenscanner" [IAI 2012]

4.2 Translation Memory Systems

When working with translation memory systems eye-tracking can be applied to evaluate the usability of different systems. There are several translation memory systems on the market. They can be divided into proprietary and open source systems. Proprietary systems are licensed under exclusive legal conditions, the rights belonging to the copyright holder. These systems can be for free or commercial. In contrast, open source systems can be used and modified by anybody since the source code is made available. The question of whether the one is better than the other or whether they are intuitively usable can be tested with eye-tracking experiments.

In a pilot study we compared the newest version of SDL Trados Studio[1] with the newest version of OmegaT[2]. Eye-tracking was carried out with a Tobii TX 300. Fixation duration and fixation count of the term window, the fuzzy match window and the source and target text windows can be found in Fig. 3 and 4. The red bar represents the results for SDL Trados, the blue ones for OmegaT.

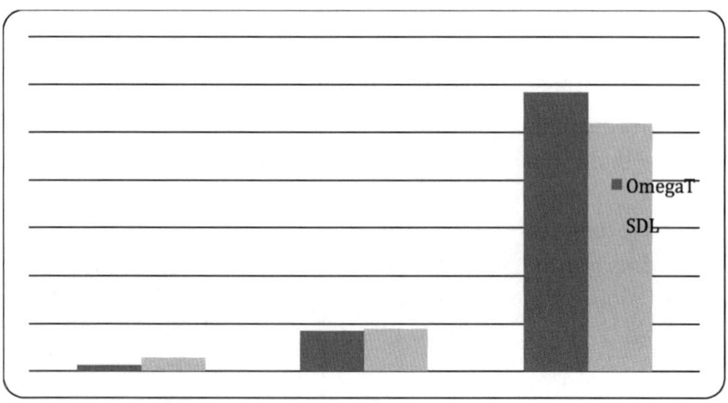

Fig. 3: Fixation duration (in seconds)

1 http://www.trados.com/

2 http://www.omegat.org/

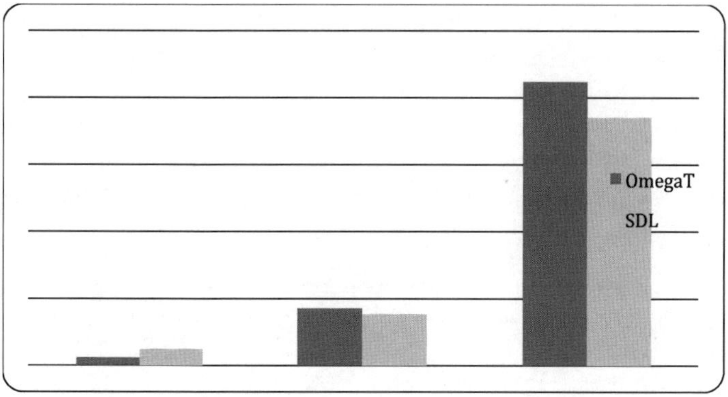

Fig. 4: *Fixation count (sum)*

The results show that fixation count and fixation duration show similar behavior. In both translation memory systems the terminology window is more or less ignored. Furthermore, the fuzzy match window does not play an important role for either translation memory system. Instead, we observe longer fixation durations as well as more fixation counts for OmegaT compared to SDL Trados. This might be an indicator, that the usability and efficiency of Trados SDL could be slightly better.

Interestingly enough, there is also space for improvement concerning the proprietary software: The heat map in Fig. 5 shows that – when working with SDL Trados – the translator looks at the source segment as well as on the target segment. The fuzzy match window, which is displayed at the top of both translation windows, is nearly neglected. This means that the user reads the suggested translation candidate in the the target text window instead of the fuzzy match window. However, the questions remain why and when the fuzzy match window is still looked at.

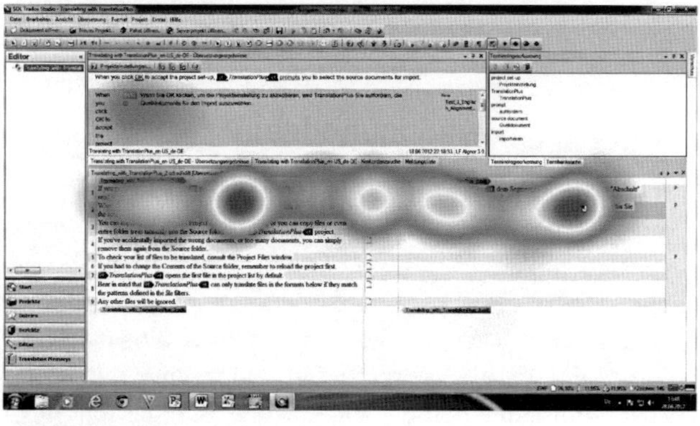

Fig. 5: *Heat map of SDL window*

The gaze plot of the same translation situation (Fig. 6) reveals that the fuzzy match window is looked at only at the very beginning of the translation process of this segment (with fixation numbers 5, 6 and 7). This can be interpreted as orientation phase. As mentioned above, in the ongoing translation process this window is completely neglected. Therefore, the benefit of the fuzzy match window is questionable – further investigations will show whether it can be omitted.

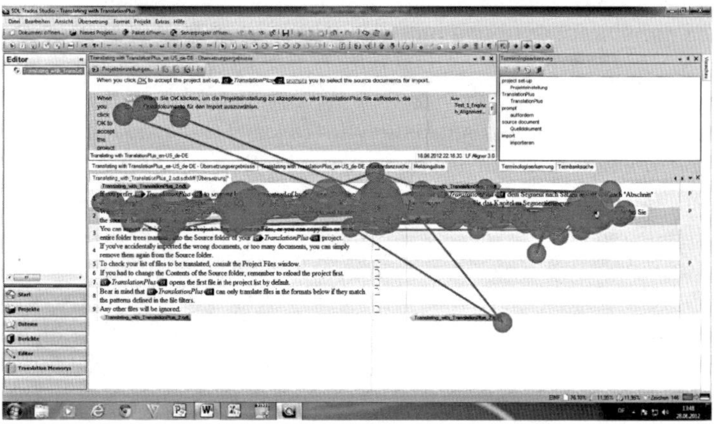

Fig. 6: *Gaze plot of SDL window*

For the translation situation displayed in Figures 5 and 6, the terminology window is completely ignored. This example corroborates the fixation duration and count in Fig. 3 and 4. Again, further research has to reveal whether this is the result of a visual (and cognitive) overload when working with translation memory systems. Gaze-induced word clouds as discussed in section 4.1 could help to resolve this overload.

4.3 Use of corpus data

The basic idea of using corpora in translator training is that a parallel corpus consists of a more comprehensive and diverse variety of source language items and possible translation solutions than a dictionary could ever display. Thus, in translator training and practice, parallel corpora are, for instance, explored for terminology look-up, for teaching the use of collocations or as translation memories. Additionally, parallel corpora can assume the role of grammatical reference works for translation training and practice. In order for corpora to serve this purpose, they need to be enriched with linguistic information (e.g. part-of-speech tagging or syntactic treebank annotation). Offering the possibility to search for word, collocations or grammatical constructions (e.g. typological differences such as clefting, raising structures), the concordances generated on the basis of parallel corpora are far more comprehensive and exhaustive (cf. S. Hansen-Schirra et al. 2012).

Combining corpus processing with gaze-assisted translation tools, we tested in a case study how corpus information is displayed when a translational problem is identified on a basis of gaze length and regression paths: We asked two translators to translate a specialised text from English into German and French. The text was taken from the user manual of Tobii Studio, the Software of the Tobii eye-trackers in the eye-tracking lab of the University Mainz/Germersheim. The eye-tracking was carried out using a Tobii TX 300. We used the eye-tracking to ad hoc build a reading model for this type of specialised translation. Problematic text passages in the source text were identified by fixation durations (3 seconds in this setting; but this could be modified) and regression paths. Fig. 7 shows that both criteria apply to the personal pronoun "we" (long fixation in line 5, regression to line 1). At this point the personal pronoun is indeed difficult to translate into German and French, because English specialised texts, especially in the area of technical documentation, are more people-oriented and less content-oriented, unlike German or French specialised texts (cf. J. House 1997). Therefore the use of personal pronouns in the English source text forms a contrastive gap and a translational problem. A literal translation into German and French would not be wrong, but unusual for the recipient. As a translational aid at this point a concordance search is started in the subcorpora of the OPUS Corpus[3], using the same text type, and the first three hits are being displayed (cf. Fig. 7). Naturally, these concordances represent only a random selection. But this way the translator gets first suggestions for possible translations. In fact for both target languages a construction using the passive voice seems a conventional strategy for the translation.

3 http://opus.lingfil.uu.se/bin/opuscqp.pl

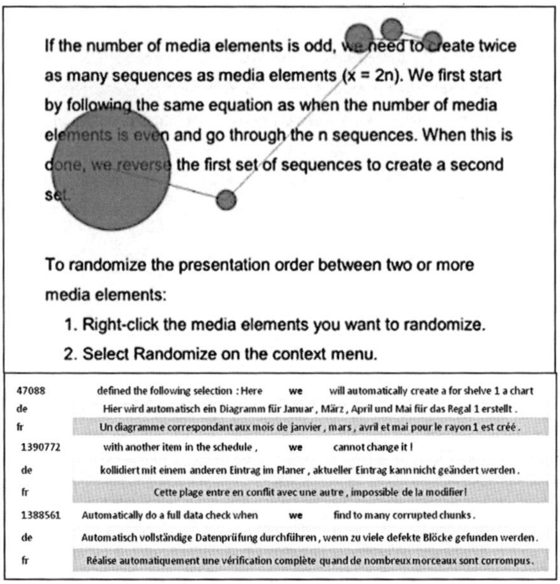

Fig. 7: Gaze-assisted translation workbench [cf. Hansen-Schirra 2012]

5. Use of gaze assisted interaction after translation

Usually, translators prefer translating a text from scratch over post-editing machine translation output. Evaluations using eye-tracking and key logging, however, show that post-editing of machine translation can be more efficient than translating highly repetitive and conventionalised texts. In our experiment 12 translators were asked to translate three texts with raising degrees of difficulty, whereas 12 translators post-edited the machine translation output of these texts. The translation and post-editing process was recorded with the key logging software Translog and with a Tobii TX 300.

Fig. 8 compares the fixation durations of the source text window of the translation (T_ST) and the post-editing (P_ST) tasks. The results show that fixation duration during translation is correlated to text complexity. The easier the text is, the lower is the fixation duration during the translation process. Instead, the degree of text complexity does not have an impact on the fixation durations for post-editing. Moreover, the post-editing task seems to be more efficient compared to the translation with respect to fixation duration (cf. S. Gutermuth/S. Hansen-Schirra 2012).

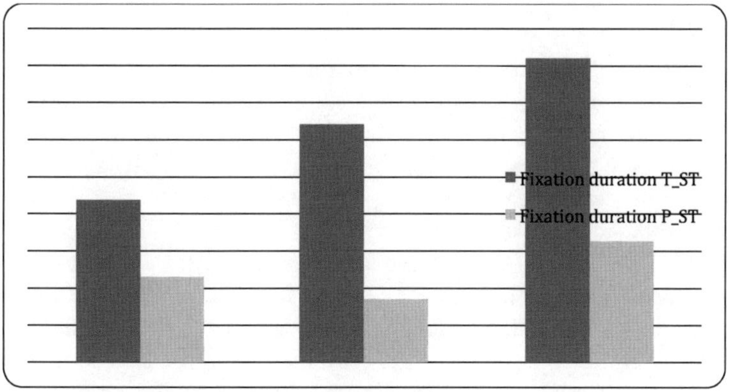

Fig. 8: *Fixation duration for post-editing vs. translation*

However, it is still unclear whether the translator evolves certain strategies when postediting the text or whether certain linguistic structures pose special problems for the processing of the machine output (e.g. contrastive gaps). The gaze plot in Fig. 9 shows that certain constructions like finite or non-finite clauses trigger the translator to look back in the source text window to check the original construction and meaning. Further research has to verify whether specific patterns can be derived from this behavior and whether gaze-enhanced corpus-based translation candidates can help to solve these problems as was suggested in section 4. This could improve teaching and practice in the area of post-editing pre-translated text.

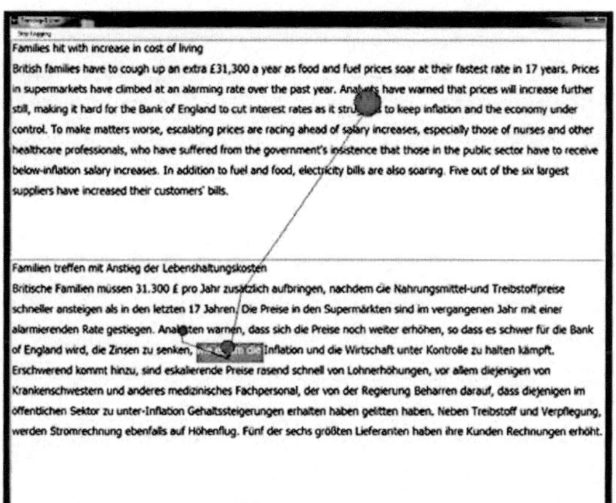

Fig. 9: *Post-editing of machine translation*

6. Conclusions

In this paper we reported on innovative concepts for the use of gaze-assisted tools and interaction in modern translational workflow. We distinguished three stages of the general process: before, during and after translation. We discussed how eye-tracking could improve the efficiency of controlled language checkers making the preparatory text processing more productive. During the translation process, terminology look-up can benefit from gaze-assisted implementations. Additionally, we have shown that evaluation through eye-tracking can improve the usability of translation memory systems. In addition, eye-tracking can be applied to detect translation problems for which gaze-enhanced tools can, in turn, provide corpus information to display translation candidates. Finally, the same holds true for the evaluation of post-editing machine translation output. The prototypes and pilot studies discussed in this paper may help improving the translation practice and the translational workflow. However, they may also offer valuable clues for translation training and education.

References

Doherty, S./ Sh. O'Brien/ C. Michael (2010): *Eye tracking as an MT evaluation technique.* In: Machine Translation. 24/1. 1-13.

Gassmann, T. (2009): *Kombination maschineller und computergestützter Übersetzungsprozesse bei Corporate Language Management der Daimler AG.* Johannes Gutenberg-Universität Mainz. Mainz (MA Thesis).

Gutermuth, S./S. Hansen-Schirra (2012): *Post-editing machine translation – a usability test for professional translation settings. Eye Track Behavior 2012*, Leuven, 9. October 2012.

Hansen-Schirra, S. (2012): Nutzbarkeit von Sprachtechnologien für die Translation. In: Transkom: Zeitschrift für Translationswissenschaft und Fachkommunikation.

Hansen-Schirra, S./ S. Neumann / E. Steiner (2012): Cross-linguistic Corpora for the Study of Translations. Insights from the Language Pair English-German. Berlin/New York.

House, J. (1997): *Translation quality assessment. A model revisited.* Tübingen.

Hyrskykari, A./ P. Majaranta/ A. Aaltonen / K.-J. Räihä (2000): Design issues of iDict: a gaze-assisted translation aid. In: In proceedings of the 2000 symposium on Eye Tracking Research and Applications [ETRA2000]. New York. 9–14.

Hyrskykari, A./ Majaranta, P./ Räihä, K.-J. (2003): *Proactive Response to Eye Movements.* In: Rauterberg/M. Menozzi/J. Wesson (eds), Proceedings of INTERACT 2003 September 1-5. Zürich. 129–136.

IAI (Institut der Gesellschaft zur Förderung der Angwandten Informationsforschung), (2009a) CLATClient Manual. 4.1

IAI (Institut der Gesellschaft zur Förderung der Angwandten Informationsforschung), (2009b) CLATIntroduction Version. 4.1

IAI (Institut der Gesellschaft zur Förderung der Angwandten Informationsforschung), (2012) DEMO-Webschnittstelle Autoindexierung sowie WordClouds.

Jakobsen, A. L. (2009): *Looking at the Eyes of Translators. Paper for the Ist International Research Workshop on Methodology in Translation Process Research. University of Graz, April 6–8*. 2009.

Lagoudaki, E. (2006): *Translation Memories Survey 2006. Translation Memory Systems: Enlightening users' perspective. Key findings of the TM Survey 2006 carried out during July and August 2006*. Imperial College London, November 2006.

Lommel, A. (2004): *LISA 2004 Translation Memory Survey. Translation Memory and Translation Memory Standards*. Edited by Rebecca Ray. Localization Industry Standards Association.

O'Brien, S. (2011): *Towards Predicting Post-Editing Productivity*. In: Machine Translation. 25/3. 197–215.

Rösener, Ch. (2010): *Computational linguistics in the translator's workflow – combining Authoring tools and Translation Memory Systems*. Proceedings of NAACL HLT 2010. CL&W – Workshop on Computational Linguistics and Writing: Writing Processes and Authoring Aids. Los Angeles, 1st – 6th June 2010.

Harnessing the Potential of Eye-Tracking for Media Accessibility

Agnieszka Szarkowska (University of Warsaw)
Izabela Krejtz (University of Social Sciences and Humanities)
Krzysztof Krejtz (University of Social Sciences and Humanities)
Andrew Duchowski (Clemson University)

Introduction

This article presents an overview of eye-tracking research studies in the area of media accessibility carried out by the Audiovisual Translation Lab at the Institute of Applied Linguistics, University of Warsaw, in cooperation with the Interdisciplinary Center for Applied Cognitive Studies at the University of Social Sciences and Humanities in Warsaw (SWPS). Media accessibility is here understood as various tools providing access to audiovisual media content for people with sensorial disabilities: in the form of subtitles for those who are deaf or hard of hearing and in the form of audio description (AD) for those who are blind or partially sighted.

The article begins with a brief discussion of various applications of eye-tracking to audiovisual translation and media accessibility, and then continues with a presentation of the following four studies carried out by the authors of this article: (1) on subtitling for the deaf and hard of hearing (SDH) as the Polish contribution to the DTV4ALL project, (2) an on-going study on SDH on digital television, (3) audio description in education, and (4) audio description in art.

1. Eye-tracking, reading and audiovisual translation

Over the last thirty years eye-tracking methodology has been successfully applied to a host of research domains (for an overview see A. Duchowski 2002, K. Rayner 1998). A rapidly growing number of studies is using eye movement behaviour to investigate individual differences in cognitive processes, most frequently in visual attention. A. Duchowski (2002) classifies the role of eye-trackers in research as either diagnostic or interactive. In the diagnostic approach we gather objective numerical data of subjects' attentional processes, whereas in the interactive studies eye movements are used as a tool allowing users to operate many applications such as eye-typing systems for disabled people who cannot type or use a mouse (e.g. P. Majaranta, K.-J. Raiha 2002). Although interactive gaze-contingent subtitles, appearing when our eyes look for them, are just a near future, in our projects we concentrated on the analysis of subtitle reading patterns across different groups of film viewers as well as on the influence of audio description on the film and artworks viewing process.

Eye-tracking has been extensively used in reading studies (see K. Rayner 1998, K. Rayner et al. 2012), particularly for the analysis of monosemiotic texts. It has been found that when reading printed text in English the eyes make quick movements (saccades) from one word to another, lasting for about 30-50 milliseconds (ms) or 7-9 letter spaces, and they stop on words, resulting in fixations, usually lasting for about 100-500 ms (K. Rayner 1998, K. Rayner et al. 2012). The duration of a fixation depends on a number of factors, such as the length of a word (longer words tend to be fixated with higher probability than shorter words), its frequency (the more frequent the word, the less likely it is to be fixated) and grammatical category (content words are fixated 85% of the time, while function words only 35%, see P.A. Carpenter, M.A. Just 1983, K. Rayner, S.A. Duffy 1988, K. Rayner 1998, K. Rayner et al. 2012).

Reading subtitles is a much more complex process than reading monosemiotic texts like a printed page with no illustrations, because along with reading the subtitles, viewers are also watching the moving images accompanied by sound. As a dynamic form of communication, film demands more cognitive resources than watching a scene and reading separately. Watching a film with subtitles combines two types of information processing with different time parameters for fixations and saccades, generally longer fixations and saccades for scenes perception and shorter for reading subtitles. The viewer is scanning a dynamically changing scene, and simultaneously s/he is tracking the text at the bottom of the screen. This is an example of a dual task causing high switching costs between scene viewing and reading subtitles for some types of viewers.

The presence or absence of sound also seems to be an important factor influencing the way we read subtitles and watch audio described films. When reading subtitles, people usually can hear the film soundtrack, which probably makes the reading different than reading printed text. It has been found that 'mean fixation durations are longer when reading aloud or while listening to a voice reading the same text than in silent reading' (A. Duchowski 2002: 2), which in fact is the case with subtitling. As an extra audio track, audio description also seems to change film viewing patterns. A recent study by A. Vilaró et al. (2012) showed that viewing patterns can be modified by changing the audio track. This result is also corroborated by our findings, reported in I. Krejtz et al. (2012).

2. Previous eye-tracking studies on subtitling

Probably the most famous and widely quoted researcher involved in eye-tracking and subtitling is G. d'Ydewalle. Together with his associates, G. d'Ydewalle examined a number of issues related to the process of reading subtitles in films, such as the automaticity of reading subtitles (G. d'Ydewalle et al. 1991), the importance of presence/absence of sound when reading subtitles (G. d'Ydewalle et al. 1987, G. d'Ydewalle, I. Gielen 1992), the influence of the number of lines on the reading process (G. d'Ydewalle 1991, G. d'Ydewalle, I. Gielen 1992, G. d'Ydewalle, W. de Bruycker 2007), the familiarity with subtitling as a factor impacting reading (d'Ydewalle et. al. 1991), the language of film dialogue vs. the language of subtitles (G. d'Ydewalle, W. de Bruycker 2007), and the reading of adults vs. children (G. d'Ydewalle, W. de Bruycker 2007). The reading of subtitles has been found to be a largely automatic process: 'reading subtitles is more or less obligatory' (G. d'Ydewalle et. al. 1991: 650), regardless of the presence/absence of sound and the (in)familiarity with subtitling. According to their findings, people who are familiar with subtitles read them fluently and effortlessly (G. d'Ydewalle/I. Gielen 1992, G. d'Ydewalle/W. de Bruycker 2007).

The eye-tracking measures examined by d'Ydewalle and his associates included the number of fixations per subtitle, fixation duration, saccade amplitude, regressions in a subtitle, subtitle skipping as well as shifts between subtitles and the video picture (see G. d'Ydewalle, W. de Bruycker 2007). The results showed that when reading film subtitles, as opposed to print, viewers tend to make more regressions than in regular reading. The fixation durations in subtitles are also shorter. As for the number of lines, the time spent in a subtitle was proportionally higher in two-line subtitles, which also contain more verbal information difficult to be inferred from the screen, than in one-liners. This prompted G. d'Ydewalle, W. de Bruycker (2007) to state that a more regular reading pattern can be found in two-liners.

G. d'Ydewalle et al. (1987) are widely quoted as having provided evidence for the famous 'six-seconds rule', according to which a two-line subtitle should appear on screen for six seconds – not less because viewers will not be able to read it, and not more because they will re-read a longer subtitle. G. d'Ydewalle et al. (1987: 321) stated: 'For subtitles with two lines the six-seconds rule appears to be excellent for our sample of subjects. In other cases, the existing 'rule of thumb' (the six-seconds rule) of most TV stations is supported by our data'. On a more critical note, it needs to be stressed that the quality of subtitles tested in the studies mentioned above was not always consistent with current subtitling standards. For instance, in G. d'Ydewalle et al. (1987), subtitles consisted of lines up to 32 characters, which is much less than the usual number now (up to 40). In the case of one-line subtitles, they were sometimes displayed in the upper line, and not, as it is usually done in professional subtitling, in the lower line (G. d'Ydewalle, W. de Bruycker 2007: 198) This may have had influence the eye-tracking results. Another major limitation of the abovementioned studies lies in the small number of participants they were based on[1] and thus in their generalizability.

A number of studies on closed captions, in Europe known as subtitles for the deaf and hard of hearing (SDH), was conducted in the US by C. Jensema and his colleagues. In C. Jensema (1998), the participants of the study (578 of whom 205 were deaf, 110 hard of hearing and 262 hearing) were shown video segments subtitled at different speeds. The most comfortable reading speed was found to be 145 wpm, but viewers did not find it difficult to adapt to subtitles of up to 170 wpm. As reported by C. Jensema (1998), frequent subtitle readers – in this case deaf and hard of hearing viewers – were more comfortable with faster subtitles. Hearing viewers, unaccustomed to watching subtitles, preferred slightly slower reading speeds. This stands in contrast with professional SDH standards in Europe, where higher subtitling rates are produced for hearing viewers and lower rates for the hearing impaired.

In another study, C. Jensema et al. (2000a) examined eye movements of six subjects when watching video clips with and without subtitles. In their seminal article they famously stated that 'the addition of captions to a video resulted in major changes in eye movement patterns, with the viewing process becoming primarily a reading process' (2000a: 275). Another major finding was that the higher the reading speed, the more time will be spent on the subtitle area (vs. the image). This result was further corroborated in the study by C. Jensema et al. (2000b), where the viewers looked at subtitles 84% of the time and only 14% at the video picture (and 2% off the video). This, of course, depends on the type of film and the amount of dialogue it contains – it is enough to compare a Woody Allen film with a typical action movie.

On the European ground, Z. de Linde and N. Kay (1999) tested 10 deaf and 10 hearing subjects, recording their eye movements when watching a number of TV programmes such as news, chat show, soap opera, comedy and documentary with intralingual English subtitles. They measured how much time the subjects took to read each word, the number and duration of deflections (jumps between the subtitle and the image), the number of regressions (i.e. re-reading of words

1 Curiously, d'Ydewalle et al. 1987 do not give the data on the number of participants. G. d'Ydewalle, W. de Bruycker (2007) tested 12 adults and 8 children; G. d'Ydewalle et al. (1991) tested 8 American and 18 Dutch students.

and characters) and re-readings of entire subtitles. The authors found a correlation between subtitles and the programme type on the grounds of 'associated discourse styles' (1999: 75), for instance chat shows, as opposed to documentaries, have higher subtitling rates, which in turn has a direct influence on reading speed, which is higher. According to Z. de Linde and N. Kay (1999: 76), 'faster subtitle rates induce faster reading speeds' and 'slow subtitles lead to more re-reading'. Among other factors influencing the reading process were the visibility of the speaker and film editing techniques, such as shot changes, which were the cause of increased re-reading of subtitles. In conclusion, the authors suggest that slow subtitles 'may be more ideal for active location shots' and faster subtitles for 'studio presentations with a static newsreader' (Z. de Linde, N. Kay 1999: 76).

E. Perego et al. (2010) analysed the cognitive processing of a subtitled film fragment based on eye-tracking data combined with word recognition and visual scene recognition. In their study, poor line segmentation in two-line subtitles did not seem to have any negative influence on subtitle comprehension. This finding goes against the results obtained by D.J. Rajendran et at. (2011), who examined the effects of text chunking on subtitling and found that 'chunking improves the viewing experience by reducing the amount of time spent reading subtitles' (2011: 1). The difference in the results may stem from the fact that E. Perego et al. (2012) examined block subtitles whereas D.J. Rajendran et a. (2011) evaluated chunking in live subtitling.

E. Ghia (2012) carried out an eye-tracking experiment testing the role of literal and non-literal translation strategies in interlingual subtitling (foreign film subtitled into subjects' mother tongue). The goal of the study was 'to help disclose the processes of cognitive mapping involved in the perception of subtitled input, and to investigate whether discrepancy of information between ST and TT is liable to affect viewers' overall watching behaviour' (2012: 164). It was found that in the case of non-literal translation strategies, the number of deflections between the subtitle and the image was higher than in the case of literal strategies. This, the author argues, may point to a divergence between the viewers' expectations of a more literal translation and the text they see in the non-literal subtitles.

S. Moran (2012) tested how word frequency and cohesion influence the cognitive effort expended when reading subtitles. Having examined different versions of the same clip (low vs. high frequency and low vs. high cohesion variables), the author reported that subjects watching high-frequency subtitles had significantly lower fixation durations on subtitles, spent more time on watching the video image and had better results in the post-eye-tracking questionnaire. In contrast, participants watching subtitles with low-frequency words and with the low-cohesion variable had to expend more processing effort to read the subtitles, as demonstrated by higher fixation durations. The results are particularly interesting given that the subtitles with low-frequency words were shorter than those with high frequency words. What is more, as pointed out by S. Moran (2012: 216), the results also 'weaken the authority of the currently practiced 6-second rule which assumes a connection between character count and reading speed/difficulty'. S. Moran (2012: 185) therefore concludes that 'a practical solution to making subtitles more readable is not in reducing the amount of text, but increasing the frequency of lexical items and their combination'.

C. Caffrey (2012) examined the effects of experimental subtitling in the form of pop-up gloss on the reception of TV anime. Pop-up gloss is a note appearing 'on screen to explain or comment on culturally marked items appearing in each of the semiotic channels' (p. 226); it usually explains culturally marked elements from Japanese culture. The analysis of four measures: (1) the percentage of skipped subtitles, (2) the percentage of gaze time in subtitles, (3) the mean fixation duration, and (4) the word fixation probability demonstrated that the presence of pop-up glosses increased the percentage of subtitle skipping, which indicated that viewers' attention was directed from reading the subtitles to looking at the gloss. What is more, participants watching the clips with both pop-up glosses and subtitles felt the subtitles were displayed at higher reading speeds than those participants who watched the clips with subtitles only – in spite of the fact that the subtitle reading speeds were the same in the two conditions. On the positive side, pop-up glosses were helpful in fostering the understanding of culture-specific elements.

To recap, previous eye-tracking studies addressed a number of interesting issues related to subtitling in general and to SDH in particular. The findings provided important insights into our knowledge on how people read subtitles. The vast majority of studies, however, was conducted on relatively small samples of subjects and focused mainly on the English language. Therefore, what is needed now is replicating some of the abovementioned studies as well as addressing new research questions. In our research on SDH reported in this article we have decided to focus on the Polish language by testing Polish hearing, hard of hearing and deaf subjects. We also examine a few recurrent themes in subtitling which have still not been resolved once and for all, such as the edited/verbatim subtitles debate and the subtitling reading speed.

3. Subtitling for the deaf and hard of hearing – the Polish contribution to the DTV4ALL project

The goal of this study was to establish European standards in subtitling for the deaf and hard of hearing, mostly by verifying participants' preferences with their cognitive system capabilities measured through eye-tracking. To address this goal, an eye-movement study was designed and conducted in Poland, Spain, England, Italy and partially in Greece and Germany. The detailed findings of the study are reported in Romero-Fresco (ed., in press). Below we present an overview of our methodology and major findings.

3.1. Rationale

When it comes to subtitling for the deaf and hard of hearing, each country cultivates its own tradition. For instance, on some Spanish TV channels sound information is placed in the top right-hand corner, while in Poland it is traditionally capitalised and situated at the bottom of the screen. Some countries, such as the US, have a long-standing tradition of verbatim subtitles, while others, Poland among them, have come a long way from extensive editing to more faithful and literal subtitles (see A. Szarkowska 2010). The DTV4ALL project addressed the different ways in which SDH is now provided in various countries with a view to creating common European SDH standards based on a number of measures, such as viewers' preferences and eye-tracking data.

3.2. The study material

The study consisted of four major components:

1. a pre-test questionnaire on SDH, where personal data on each participant was gathered;
2. film material of 23 clips, divided into nine parameters (e.g. character identification), each testing three or two independent variables (e.g. colours, speaker-dependent placement and tags);
3. three comprehension questions after each clip; the first one about general understanding, the second about the textual content of subtitles and the third about visual elements in the clip;
4. a post-eye-tracking survey on participants' preferences concerning particular subtitling solutions.

The following subtitling parameters, comprising the existing SDH solutions and the ones which could potentially be implemented in the future, were tested in the study:

1. Character ID (colours, speaker-dependent placement, name tags)
2. Subtitling style (verbatim, standard, edited)
3. Position (top, bottom, mixed)
4. Emotions (verbal description, smileys, no description)
5. Sounds (verbal description, icons, no description)
6. Justification (centre, left-aligned)
7. Borders (borders around subtitle letters, no borders)
8. Boxes (black box around subtitles, no black box)
9. Shadows (shadows around subtitle letters, no shadows).

The clips, each lasting about one minute, were taken from the *Shrek* trilogy, dubbed into Polish, so the subtitles tested were in fact intralingual (i.e. based on the translated Polish dialogue).

Thanks to the different ways of collecting data (preference questionnaires, eye-tracking data, comprehension questions) we hoped to obtain information on which parameters were optimal for SDH and which could be recommended for further implementation in digital television. Since in this article our major focus is on eye-tracking, below we report data on the eye-tracking tests.

3.3. Participants

The total number of participants in the eye-tracking tests in Poland was 40. They were divided into three groups based on their degree of hearing loss: (1) the deaf, (2) the hard of hearing and (3) the hearing (the control group).

Age group	Deaf	Hard of hearing	Hearing
15-24	1	5	3
25-39	7	9	4
40-59	1	2	2
60+	0	5	1
Total	9	21	10

Table 1. Participants by age and hearing loss

There was a comparable number of male and female participants (46% vs. 54% respectively).

3.4. Procedure

Eye movements were recorded with an EyeLink CL eye-tracking system (SR Research Ltd.). The EyeLink system uses infrared, video-based technology to compute the distance between the pupil centre and corneal reflection. Signals were generated by the eye-tracker at a frequency rate of 500 Hz when a stable corneal reflection was obtainable from a participant. Stimuli were presented on a 17-inch LCD colour monitor with 60 Hz refresh rate. Participants were seated in a chair in front of the monitor positioned at an eye level at a viewing distance of approximately 60 cm, maintained by a forehead and chin-rest.

Participants were presented with 23 clips (each lasting about 1 minute) during which their eye movements were recorded. After three or two clips (i.e. one parameter), participants answered additional three paper and pencil questions concerning their subtitle preferences. Then it was followed by recalibration. Drift corrections were performed before each trial.

Eye-tracking data were analysed for fixations and saccades using the Eyelink DataViewer (SR Research Ltd). For each trial, areas of interest (AOI) were drawn based on prior hypotheses. We compared mean reading time and time to first fixation to the AOIs. For the behavioural data, the percentage of correct answers to comprehension questions was calculated.

Time to first fixation was calculated in milliseconds (ms) and defined as the time which elapsed between subtitle onset and the first fixation that entered the AOI with subtitles. Thus, time to first fixation reflected how much time after the subtitle onset it took the participants to look at the subtitle AOI.

Mean reading time was defined as the period of time that participants spent on reading subtitles compared to the time spent on watching the whole clip. We calculated mean dwell time, i.e. the sum of durations of all the fixations, in the subtitle AOI and compared it to the dwell time of all fixations across the whole clip.

3.5. Results

The study brought about a number of interesting findings. To begin with, we observed differences in reading patterns between deaf, hard of hearing and hearing participants. For instance, hearing people tended to move their eyes from the screen to the new subtitle when a new subtitle appeared, whereas deaf people spent more time in the subtitle area, as if waiting for new subtitles to appear.

According to C. Jensema et al. (2000a: 284), 'there appears to be a general tendency to start by looking at the middle of the screen and then moving the gaze to the beginning of a caption within a fraction of a second. Viewers read the caption and then glance at the video action after they finish reading'. This regular pattern, the authors argue, is repeated when another subtitle caption appears. In our study, it was more common in the case of deaf participants (see Fig. 1).

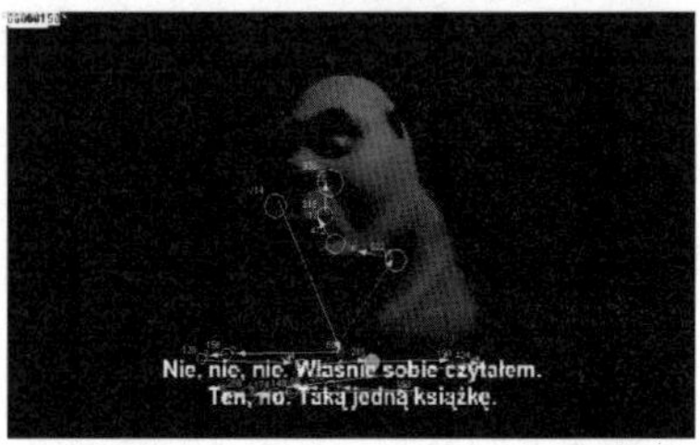

Fig. 1: *Gaze plot of the reading pattern of a deaf participant when reading verbatim subtitles*

Generally, however, the process of reading subtitles in our study was not as linear and regular as C. Jensema et al. (2000a) suggest. When reading subtitles, all the participants made quite a few jumps (called *deflections*, after Z. de Linde and N. Kay 1999) between the image and the subtitle area. On average, they switched more than six times between the image and the subtitle during its presentation, particularly in the case of two-line subtitles (see Fig. 2).

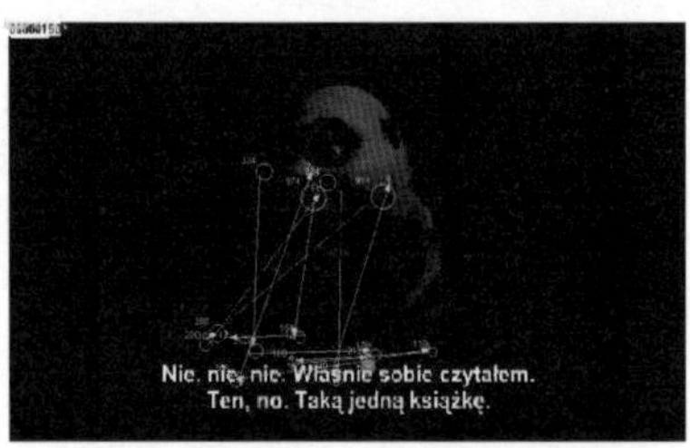

Fig. 2: *Gaze plot of the reading pattern of a hard of hearing participant when reading verbatim subtitles*

Interesting differences were observed between participants when reading three different types of subtitles: edited, standard and verbatim (Table 2). In our study, verbatim subtitles included every single word from the dialogue, even the words which are usually omitted in subtitling, such as elements of spoken language like vocatives, repetitions, false starts. In contrast, standard subtitles contained most information from the dialogue, but without the elements of oral discourse. Edited subtitles were the ones whose text was simplified and reduced: more complex syntactic structures were shortened, difficult and infrequent words were substituted with their simpler synonyms, while elements of spoken language were removed. Verbatim subtitles had shortest display times and higher reading speed, while edited subtitles were displayed at lower reading speed.

	Edited	Standard	Verbatim
Deaf	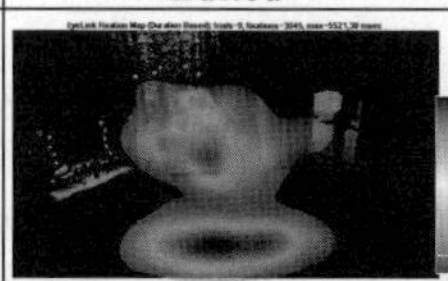	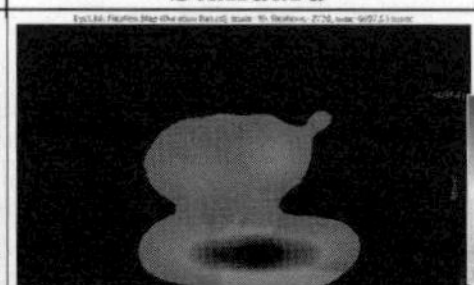	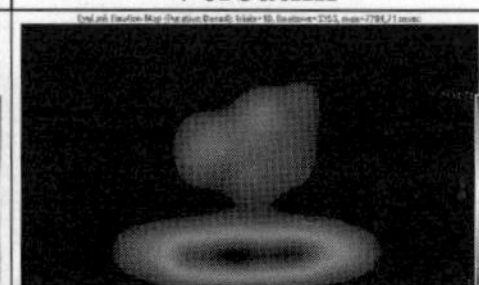
Hard of hearing	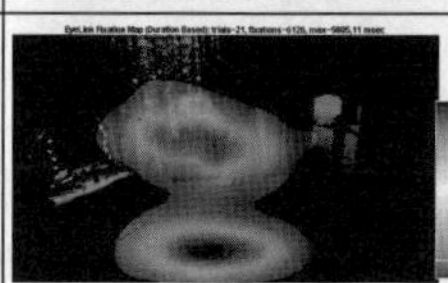	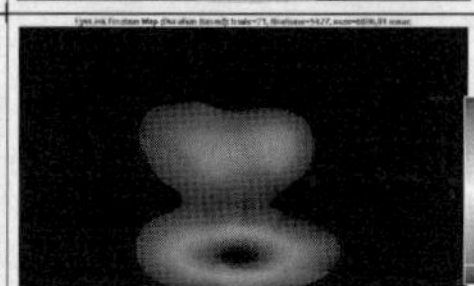	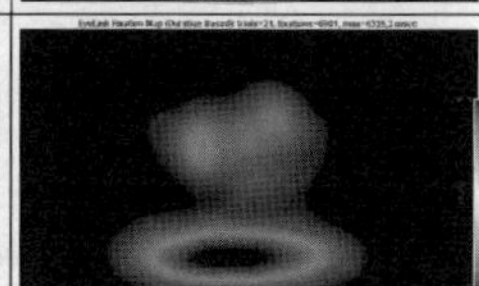
Hearing	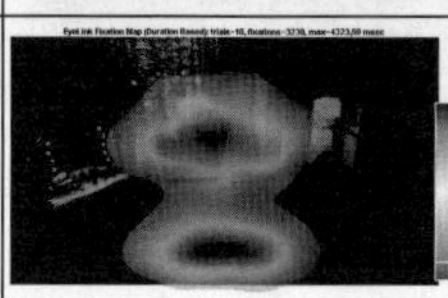	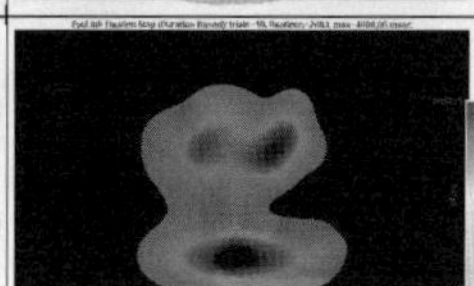	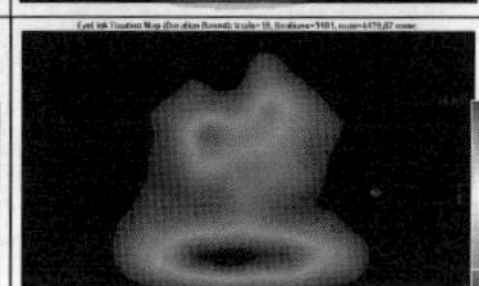

Table 2. Time spent viewing different types of subtitles

Two regular patterns can be discerned when looking at the heat maps in Table 2. First, in comparison with verbatim subtitles, edited captions induced fewer fixations on the subtitles area and more on the video image than verbatim subtitles. This means that edited subtitles allowed viewers to look more at the video picture, whereas with verbatim subtitles people spent more time in the subtitle area, thus having less time to look at the rest of the screen. Second, there is a marked difference between the three groups of participants: hearing people look more at the image and less at the subtitles, as opposed to hearing-impaired people, who spend more time in the subtitle area. In our study, hearing participants made significantly fewer fixations per subtitle (6.58) than deaf participants (8.72) (see A. Szarkowska et. al 2011 for details). This may be taken as an indication that hearing people are faster readers. It also points to the fact that reading patterns are largely affected by the subtitle reading speed.

Contrary to our initial hypotheses, whereby we expected edited captions to render highest comprehension scores, it was with verbatim subtitles that participants achieved best comprehension results. This, we acknowledge, may be attributable not only to the caption type, but also to the difficulty of the clips and particular questions, so we are far from generalising this result and we believe further tests are needed to examine this area more closely. More information on the results of this study can be found in A. Szarkowska et al. (2011).

The DTV4ALL also tested solutions that are not in common use in the subtitling profession, such as the use of smileys to denote emotions (see Fig. 3) and the use of icons to describe sounds (see Fig. 4), with a view to finding out whether target viewers would like to see them implemented in the future.

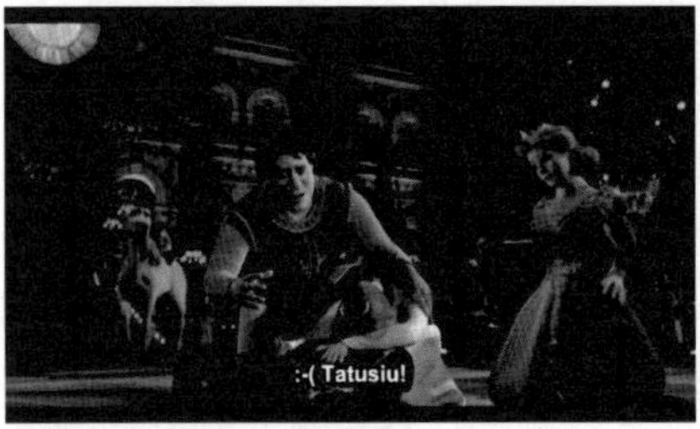

Fig. 3: A sample subtitle with a smiley denoting sadness

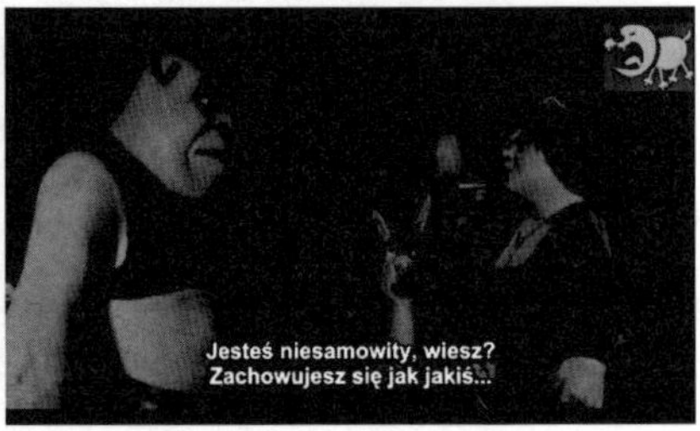

Fig. 4: An icon of a barking dog used to describe the sound

In the preferences questionnaire, none of the participants selected the smileys as their preferred option of describing emotions and only one hard of hearing viewer opted for icons as the best option of describing sounds. Eye-tracking tests showed that it took people a long time to spot the icon and that many participants did not notice the dog at all. This, of course, may be attributed to the fact that the viewers are not accustomed to such solution of describing sounds. Some other people stated they thought the dog was part of the film. Other reasons may include the quality of the picture and its placement in the top right-hand corner instead of next to subtitles. To sum up, most participants opted for verbal description as the best way of rendering sounds. As for emotions, most people preferred not to have any description, stating that emotions can be easily inferred from the image and context.

All in all, we need to note that in the case of this particular research study it was difficult to draw general conclusions because a large amount of eye-tracking data, comprehension scores and preference tests were frequently contradictory. For example, viewers tended to prefer other options than those which yielded highest comprehension scores or best eye-tracking results. What is more, viewers in different countries had different opinions as to their preferred options. Since there were many questions that remained unanswered, we decided to carry out another eye-tracking study on subtitling for the deaf and hard of hearing, this time focusing in greater detail on the question of reading speed, the editing of subtitles and differences in reading between various film genres.

4. Subtitling for the deaf and hard of hearing on digital television[2]

The goal of this on-going study is to examine the reading process of verbatim and edited subtitles among people with hearing impairments acquired at the pre-, peri- and post-lingually as well as among hearing people (the control group). The study material consists of both Polish and foreign productions. The genres examined include feature films, TV series, documentaries and news programmes.

4.1. Rationale

Since the previous study, conducted under the auspices of DTV4ALL, did not produce conclusive results on some of the most important issues related to SDH, we decided to investigate them further in more detail. The present study focuses on the questions of optimal reading speed (the two speeds tested are 12 vs. 15 cps[3]), subtitle editing (verbatim vs. edited), the influence of the film language and the film genre on the process of reading subtitles by hearing, hard of hearing and deaf viewers. Other research questions we intend to examine include the reading of content vs. grammar words, the influence of line segmentation on reading patterns, and the influence of shot changes on the re-reading of subtitles.

4.2. Participants

So far we have tested over 130 people with various degrees of hearing impairment as well as hearing people. Since this is an on-going study, the exact data on all the participants will be reported elsewhere.

4.3. Stimuli

Participants watch one of the two sets of clips (see Table 3) from five groups of materials: Polish feature films/TV series, foreign[4] feature films, Polish documentary, foreign documentary and Polish news programmes. The two sets differ in the reading speeds of subtitles; each clip is displayed with the speed of either 12 cps or 15 cps.

---

2 This study is supported by research grant No. IP2011 053471 from the Polish Ministry of Science and Higher Education for the years 2011-2013.

3 Characters per second

4 'Foreign' here means English-speaking.

The clips subtitled at the speed of 15 cps contain a verbatim version of the dialogue while those subtitled at the speed of 12 cps are edited, i.e. some linguistic structures have been simplified and elements of spoken language removed.

	Version 1	**Version 2**
1. **Polish feature film**		
Bitwa warszawska 1920 r.	12 cps	15 cps
Sami swoi	15 cps	12 cps
Londyńczycy	12 cps	15 cps
2. **Foreign feature film**		
Annie Hall	15 cps	12 cps
King's speech	12 cps	15 cps
Love actually	15 cps	12 cps
3. **Polish documentary**		
Największe cuda przyrody[5]	12 cps	15 cps
Polskie państwo podziemne	15 cps	12 cps
4. **Foreign documentary**		
Super Size Me	15 cps	12 cps
Roman Polański: Wanted and Desired	12 cps	15 cps
5. **News programme**		
Teleexpress	15 cps	12 cps
Wiadomości	12 cps	15 cps
Fakty	15 cps	12 cps

Table 3. Two sets of subtitled material

4.4. Procedure

Eye movements are recorded with SMI Red at the sampling frequency of 120 Hz. Participants are seated in front of a monitor at a distance of ca. 60 cm. After signing an informed consent to participate in the study, the participants answer a few personal questions displayed on the monitor, regarding their age, degree of

5 The original language of the film is English and its original title is *Great Natural Wonders of the World.* It is treated here, however, as a Polish film because the original voice was removed and only the Polish voice artist can be heard.

hearing loss, hearing aid/implant, education, language of daily communication, and fluency in English.

5. Eye-tracking and audio description

Apart from using eye-tracking to research subtitling for the deaf and hard of hearing, we have also examined its application to audio description. AD is a special description of what is taking place on the screen, originally created for blind and partially sighted viewers. Our recent studies have demonstrated the potential of using AD in the education of blind and partially sighted children (A. Walczak 2010, A. Walczak, A. Szarkowska (forthcoming)). Taking advantage of eye-tracking, we also studied the applicability of AD to the education of sighted children (I. Krejtz et. al 2012, K. Krejtz et al. 2012). In the remaining part of the article we first examine previous eye-tracking studies on AD and then report on the results of our eye-tracking research on AD in the education of sighted children (for more details see I. Krejtz et. al 2012, K. Krejtz et al. 2012) and AD in arts.

While there has been quite a number of studies using eye-tracking methodology to study subtitling, there are not so many on eye-tracking and audio description. A large-scale research on AD was carried out within the framework of the European DTV4ALL project (see A. Chmiel, I. Mazur 2012, I. Mazur, A. Chmiel 2012). The goal of the project was to establish European AD guidelines and address cross-cultural and cross-linguistic differences in various EU states. Most of the study was based on the Pear Tree Project (see the Special Issue of *Perspectives: Studies in Translatology* vol. 20 no.1, 2012).

Another smaller eye-tracking study was conducted by the team involved in DTV4ALL. It examined perceptions of sighted students from Poland, Italy and Spain watching short video segments from *Marie Antoinette* and then compared them with the existing English AD (see A. Chmiel et al. 2010). It turned out that the participants' gaze did not always coincide with the AD script. I. Mazur and A. Chmiel continue looking into *Marie Antoinette* in their own project on 'Eye-tracking in audio description: perception of sighted viewers and its reflection in film descriptions for the blind', funded by the Polish Ministry of Science and Higher Education (see I. Mazur, A. Chmiel 2011).

A recent study by A. Vilaró et al. (2012) addressed the question whether – and if so, how – the soundtrack influences the perception and understanding of audiovisual texts. In their experiment, they tested four different soundtracks to the same clip (*Pear Film*), comparing differences in scanpaths between viewers. The study demonstrated that the addition of sound does influence visual perception and eye movements.

Vilaró and Orero (forthcoming) examined the topic of leifmotifs, or recurrent themes, in audio description. They compared eye-tracking data with comprehension tests of a group of sighted volunteers who watched film fragments with and without AD. As predicted, people who watched the clips without AD did not notice an important detail (here a halo over the cockerel's head in the Pathé logo), as opposed to those who watched the audio described clip. A similar experiment was conducted by Orero and Vilaró (forthcoming), who looked into the question whether minute but important details regarding film characters match the participants' eye gaze and should be audio described. Participants watched three film excerpts, which were followed by questionnaires. The results showed an agreement between where the participants looked and what was audio described.

In a study on making meaning in AVT, J.-L. Kruger (2012: 67) attempted to 'correlate eye-tracking data […] with viewer constructions of the narrative'. Basing on recordings of eye movement data from Wallace Chafe's 1975 *Pear Film* combined with post-test written accounts, Kruger examined how viewers 'make sense of narrative sequences' (*ibid.*). In the eye-tracking experiment, he analysed dwell time, glance count and fixation count on objects marked with dynamic AOIs, i.e. adjusting the shape and size of the objects every few frames along with their movements in the film changing over time. The findings of the experiment suggest that 'visually peripheral elements that play a covert, top-down role in the narrative (i.e. with a higher degree of narrative salience) gain particular narrative importance when competing with the more overt, bottom-up aspects of the narrative (with an equally high narrative salience, as well as a high visual salience)' (J.-L. Kruger 2012: 67).

6. Audio description in education

Audio description is usually targeted at people who are blind or visually impaired. These viewers, as demonstrated by a number of previous studies, greatly benefit from the addition of AD to audiovisual materials. For example, an interesting study by G. Frazier and I. Coutinhoo-Johnson (1995) compared the comprehension of a video among visually impaired and sighted students. It was found that the visually impaired students who watched the audio described video had similar comprehension scores to sighted students and significantly better scores to those visually impaired students who saw the video without AD. This finding was corroborated by E. Peli, E.N. Fine and A.T. Labianca (1996), who found that visually impaired participants watching an audio described video performed better in comprehension tests than sighted participants and those visually impaired who saw the video without AD. Another experiment by

E. Schmeidler and C. Kirchner (2001), which tested comprehension among blind people watching a scientific programme with and without AD, confirmed that those participants who watched the programme with AD retained more information than those who did not hear audio description.

6.1 Rationale

The research on the possibility of adding AD to educational materials was conducted by A. Walczak (2010) and A. Walczak, A. Szarkowska (forthcoming), demonstrating promising results. Our recent studies have shown that blind and visually impaired children can benefit from audio described material. Encouraged by these findings, we decided to examine the plausibility of using AD in the education of sighted children. We hypothesised that AD can foster children's comprehension and guide their attention to what is most relevant on screen. AD could thus be used as another educational tool and a supplement to traditional education.

When watching static images, people first tend to explore the image with long saccades and shorter fixations; after a few seconds the saccade amplitude drops and fixations become longer (see D.E. Irwin, G.J. Zelinsky 2002, B.M. Velichkovsky et al. 2005). This pattern can be attributed to two modes of acquiring information: exploration and inspection. The former is used to explore the visual field in order to select a target, and the latter to inspect the target in greater detail. This division corresponds to what has been known in literature as the distinction between focal ambient (C.B. Trevarthen 1968). When watching dynamic scenes, such as films, the two modes may interplay with each other as scenes change over time.

In this study, we hypothesised that the addition of AD to the film will result in modifying children's eye movements, guiding children's visual attention, which would be reflected in a larger number of fixations, longer fixations and shorter saccades. This could indicate a more focused watching experience, resulting in better comprehension of educational content.

6.2. Participants

We tested a group of 44 primary school children aged 8-9, who watched an educational film with and without AD. Owing to poor calibration results, data from three participants were removed, giving the total of 41 participants (21 girls and 20 boys). Written consents to take part in the study were obtained from both the parents and the children. After the test, each child was rewarded with a Lego figure.

6.3. Stimuli

Children watched two 2-minute videos from the episode 'Blood' from the educational series *Once upon a time... Blood.* The experimental group watched the videos with text-to-speech audio description (for more on TTS AD see A. Szarkowska 2011).

There were two types of audio description used in the clips: synchronised and foreshadowed. Synchronised AD is the one that appears simultaneously with the action taking place on the screen. Foreshadowed AD precedes the action because when the action takes place, it is impossible to insert the description owing to the presence of dialogue (the major rule in AD is not to talk over the dialogue).

6.4. Procedure

Before the tests, the children made a lab tour and were shown the eye-tracker. They could also see how their eyes were monitored on the experimenter's screen. During the tests, children's eye movements were recorded with SR Research Ltd.'s Eye-Link CL eye-tracking system at 250 Hz. Children were seated at a distance of approx. 60 cm in front of a 17-inch LCD monitor.

Given that we were testing children and that we wanted the viewing to resemble natural conditions, we decided against using a chinrest. In consequence, we used the eye-tracker's remote mode of tracking, which requires adhesion of a contrasting dot to the participant's forehead to correct for their head movements. To facilitate calibration, we asked the children to 'shoot with their eyes' at the dots appearing on the screen.

Children were randomly assigned to two groups watching video with (the experimental group) or without AD (the control group). The experimental group was shown two 2-minute clips with AD, whereas the control group watched the same clips without AD. After watching each clip, children were presented with a scene recognition test: we showed them five pairs of pictures, where in each pair one picture was taken from the fragment they had seen and the other from another fragment of the film. Children's task was to indicate which picture they had seen in the film.

6.5. Results

In analysing data, we looked at fixation duration, fixation count and saccade amplitude. We also observed differences in the two types of AD (synchronised and foreshadowed).

A three-way mixed ANOVA analysis showed significant interaction effect between the experimental/control group, synchronised/foreshadowed AD and gender. In the experimental group during foreshadowed AD mean fixation duration was significantly longer (*M=413.04, SD=117.85*) than during synchronised AD (*M=356.04, SD=68.57*). Longer fixations may have resulted from listening to AD and anticipating the action about to happen. No significant differences in the control group were observed.

Another significant interaction was that between group and gender: it was boys' eye movements that were more influenced by AD than girls'. When watching the audio described clips, boys from the experimental group had longer fixations than boys from the control group. This may demonstrate a more focal attentional processing.

In order to verify whether children were actually looking at the parts of the video being described in AD, we also calculated fixation count in the specific areas of interest (AOI). For instance, one AOI was drawn around viruses which appeared in AD and were signalled by AD as follows: 'Suddenly, yellow crawling creatures – viruses – appear'. We analysed the period of two seconds starting with the moment the viruses appeared on screen (see Fig. 5).

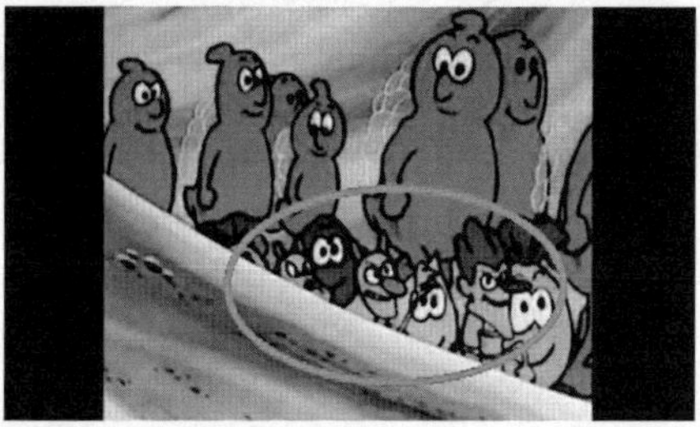

Fig. 5 *Area of interest on viruses described in AD*

In line with our predictions, it turned out that children in the experimental group had significantly more fixations on viruses (*M = 4.0, SD = 1.22*) than children from the control group (*M = 3.13, SD = 1.34*). This confirmed our hypothesis that AD guides children's attention to relevant elements of the scenes. As explained by Krejtz I. et. al. (2012), 'children followed virus movements more closely once a meaning was assigned to their creature representations'.

After eye-tracking tests, we asked the children to do a scene recognition test, where they had to choose which picture from each pair appeared in the clip they had seen (see Fig. 6).

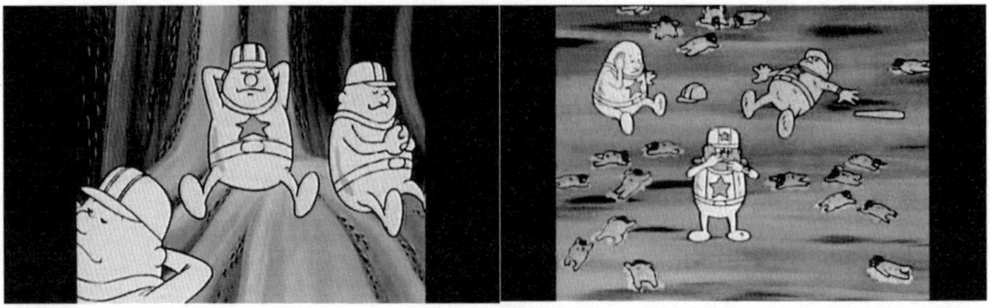

Fig. 6 *A sample pair of pictures from the scene recognition test*

Both groups reached nearly 100% correctness on this task and no significant differences were observed between conditions. However, when analysing answers to open-ended questions asked after the test during individual debriefing, we observed interesting results regarding the use of specialised vocabulary. The use of specialised terms was tested by asking children about mitosis, the role of antibodies and who attacked the organism (see Fig. 7).

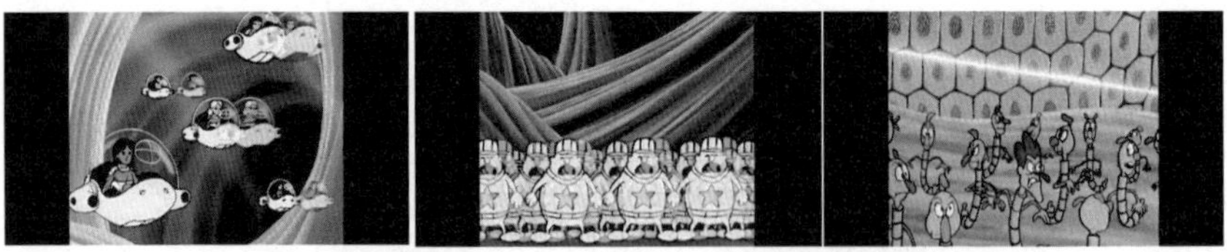

Fig. 7: *Film stills showing the mitosis of white cells (picture 1 and 2) and viruses who attached the organism (picture 3)*

Their answers were coded on a 5-point scale, where 0 stood for none, 1: wrong, 2: poor, 3: good, 4: very good. Very few children said they couldn't remember the answers or who gave incorrect answers (23.8% in the control group and 14.3% in the AD group). We then examined the answers ranked as good or very good, the difference being whether a specialised term was used or not. There was a significant correlation between the group (experimental/control) and the answer. Over 70% of children from the experimental group used specialised terms as opposed to nearly 30% of children from the control group. Table 4 presents samples of debriefing interviews, one from the experimental group and one from the control group[6].

6 Translated from Polish by A. Sz.

Experimental group	Control group
R: OK, tell me now, do you remember who copied themselves... got replicated? *G: White cells and these... ships.* *R: Alright. And what did antibodies do?* *G: Antibodies did... they... scared away the... they crawled over the viruses and as if they started to melt, something like that.* *R: OK, now, and who attacked the organism?* *G: Viruses.* *R: Great, and what is mitosis?* *G: Dividing into twos.* *R: Fantastic, thank you very much.*	*R: Alright, tell me if you remember who copied themselves?* *G: White cells and girls in ships copied themselves.* *R: Great, and what do antibodies do?* *G: Antibodies... which ones were antibodies?* *R: Well, what do you remember... do you remember which of them were the antibodies?* *G: No.* *R: OK, it doesn't matter. And do you remember who attacked the organism?* *G: The organism was attacked by the... the sticks.* *R: Uhm.* *G: The brown sticks, I don't know what they're called.* *R: Ok, it's alright. And what is mitosis?* *G: I have no clue.* *R: Good, that's all.*

Table 4. *Sample post-eye-tracking test interviews with two girls: (1) from the experimental and (2) the control group, R = researcher, G = girl*

To sum up, the findings of our study show that children's eye movements – and thus their attention – can be positively affected by AD, which helps them to focus on relevant elements of the screen. The AD script also provides children with specialised vocabulary presented in context, which fosters their understanding of educational material and facilities knowledge acquisition.

7. Audio description in art

Apart from standard audio guides for sighted viewers, more and more museums and art galleries are offering audio description for the blind and partially sighted visitors. Such description usually includes standard information like the name of the artist, the title of the painting/artwork, date, dimensions (height/width), technique as well as a verbal description of the visual aspects of the work. Following the tenets of universal design theory, according to which a product/service should be designed from conception to include as many potential and differently abled users as possible (see J.-P. Udo, D.I. Fels 2009: 1), 'exhibit designers are increasingly combining standard audio tours with audio descriptions, an 'all-in-one' concept' (ADP Standards 2009: 28). In consequence, both sighted and visually impaired people can receive the same audio description. As reported in ADP Standards (*ibid.*), sighted visitors also benefit from extended verbal descriptions of artworks. Such audio description can also be used in education as an aid to visual literacy.

This new application of audio description poses new research questions and opens new research avenues. Below we look at one such area regarding the perception of artworks – with and without audio description – by sighted students. The aim of the study was to examine the influence of audio description on perception of art among sighted young people.

Our hypothesis was that AD can precisely guide attention to the most relevant parts of the painting enabling better understanding of an artwork and fostering visual memory of the painting. AD can thus help viewers acquire new information such as specialized history about particular piece of art, promoting more elaborated information processing and stimulating their visual memory.

7.1. Participants

All participants (N=59) were students of the first two years of high school profiled towards mathematics and computer science. There were 22 male and 27 female participants.

7.2. Experimental design

The present research was a 3 (type of presentation) x 2 (order of presentation) experiment. The type of presentation was a between-subject factor. Each participant was randomly assigned to one of the three experimental conditions (types of presentation): (1) the AD group: visualization of art piece with auditory description accompanying the picture, (2) the text group: visualization of art piece with textual description presented next to the picture, (3) the control group: visualization of art piece without any description. The order of presentation was a within-subject factor. Each participant saw two paintings in random order.

7.3. Stimuli

Participants were shown two short video clips each with a still picture of two famous paintings: *The Umbrellas* by Pierre-August Renoir and *The calling of St. Matthew* by Caravaggio. The first clip lasted for 4 min and 18 sec. and the second one for 4 min. 35 sec.

In all experimental conditions we presented the students with a still image of the painting situated on the left-hand side of the screen. The experimental conditions differed in what was presented on the right-hand side of the screen. In the AD condition, the AD script was read by a voice talent (previously recorded in a studio), so the participants did not see the text, and the space on the right of the screen was left blank (see Fig. 8a). In the text condition, the script was presented in the textual form next to the picture (see Fig. 8b). In the control condition, the space on the right was again left empty (see Fig. 8c).

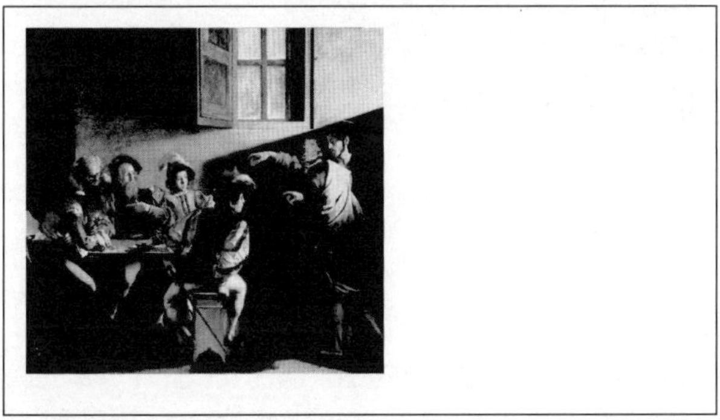

Fig. 8a. *A sample scene from the video clip presenting the Caravaggio painting in the AD condition*

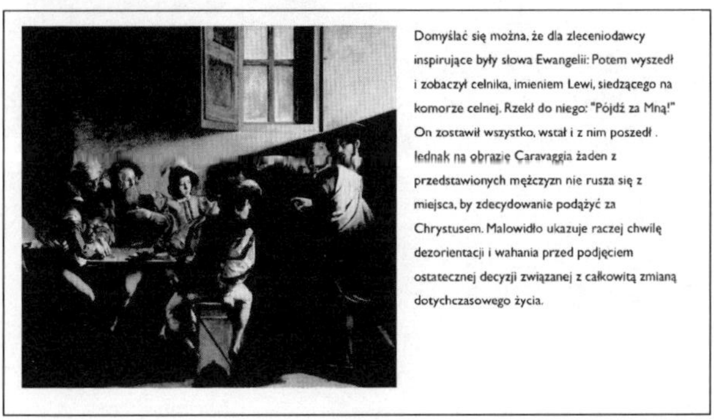

Fig. 8b: *A sample scene from the video clip presenting the Caravaggio painting in the text condition*

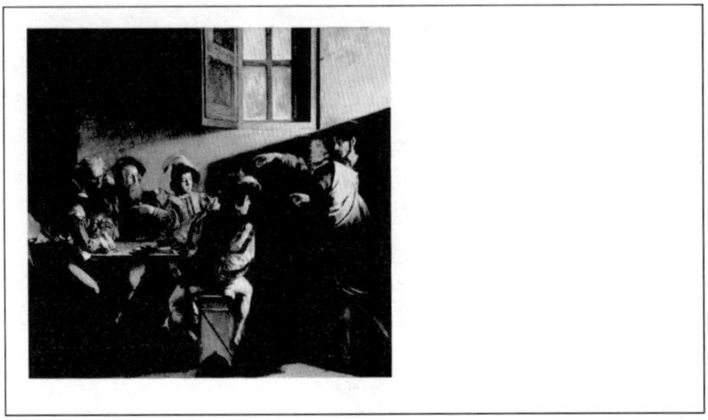

Fig. 8c: *A sample scene from the video clip presenting the Caravaggio painting in the control condition*

7.4. Apparatus

Eye movements were recorded at 250 Hz with the SMI eye-tracking system. Participants were seated in front of a computer monitor (1024 x 768 resolution; 22-inch LCD, 60 Hz refresh rate). The eye-tracker's remote mode of tracking was used to promote participants' comfort and ensure natural viewing conditions. The spatial resolution of used eye-tracking system was 0.03 degrees and gaze position accuracy 0.4 degrees. The SMI Experiment Center software was used to present stimuli and synchronize them with eye movements recorded. For fixations and saccades detection as well raw data cleaning, SMI BeGaze software was employed. We used default BeGaze settings for detecting fixations and saccades with the High Speed Event Detection method. With this method saccades are treated as primary events and fixations are derived from them. In order to capture saccades, the method uses a velocity-based algorithm. With this algorithm peak velocity threshold is set to 40 degrees per second and minimum saccade duration is set to 22 ms while minimum fixation duration is set to 50 ms.

7.5. Procedure

The experiment was conducted individually. First, each participant signed an informed consent; being underage, students were also obliged to provide a signed consent form from their parents. Then the 9-point calibration was performed. After a successful calibration procedure, two video clips with the paintings of Caravaggio and Renoir were presented in random order. After each video clip, participants were asked to solve interactive jigsaw puzzles[7] made from the painting they had just seen (see Fig. 9).

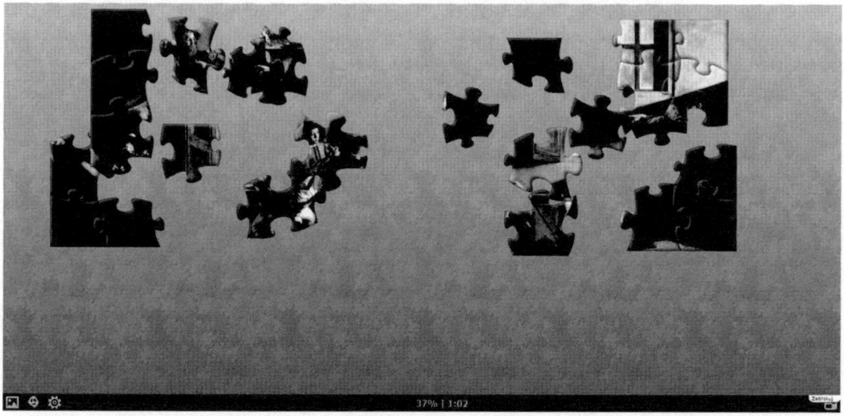

Fig. 9: Interactive jigsaw puzzle from Caravaggio's painting

After watching both video clips, participants answered a series of interactive questions on what they have learned from video clips about the painters and the works of art.

7.6. Results

A qualitative analysis of scanpaths in the AD and the control group clearly presents different viewing patterns (see Figures 10 and 11). As the AD group was closely following the audio description, they were more focused on the parts of the painting mentioned (e.g. the young man counting money at the table). In contrast, the control group is concentrated on faces, which is a typical viewing pattern, well-established in eye-tracking research, confirming that human face is a special stimulus always attracting our attention (see A. L. Yarbus 1967, O. Hershler, S. Hochstein 2005, S. R. H. Langton et al. 2008).

7 www.jigsawplanet.com

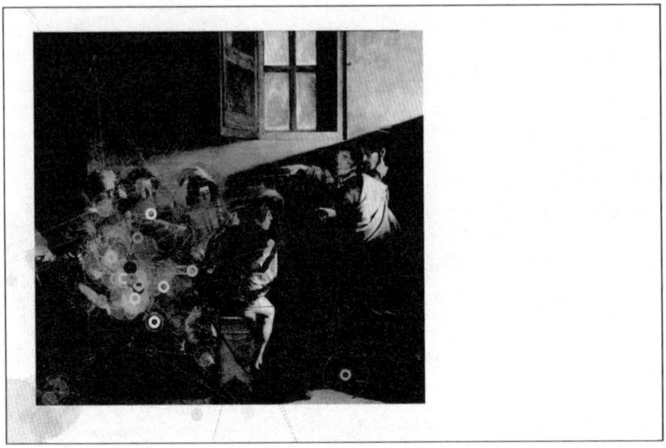

Fig. 10: *Two-second long scanpath in the AD group*

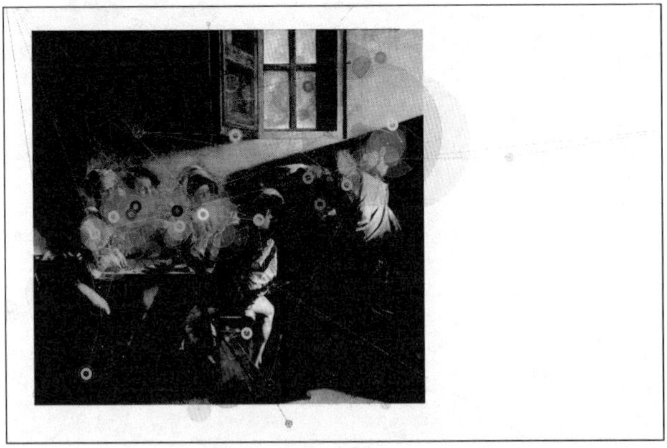

Fig. 11: *Two-second long scanpath in the control group*

To verify the influence of AD on the perception of paintings, we conducted a one-way between-subject analysis of variance, with group as the independent factor and percent of dwell time on the painting as a dependent variable. The analysis revealed a significant main effect of the experimental condition, $F(2,55) = 104.51$, $p < 0.001$. As expected, the AD group examined the painting significantly longer ($M = 76.91$; $SD = 10.73$) than the control group ($M = 60.99$, $SD = 9.73$) and the group with written text presented next of the painting ($M = 29.17$, $SD = 10.10$). The differences between all three conditions were statistically significant (see Fig. 12).

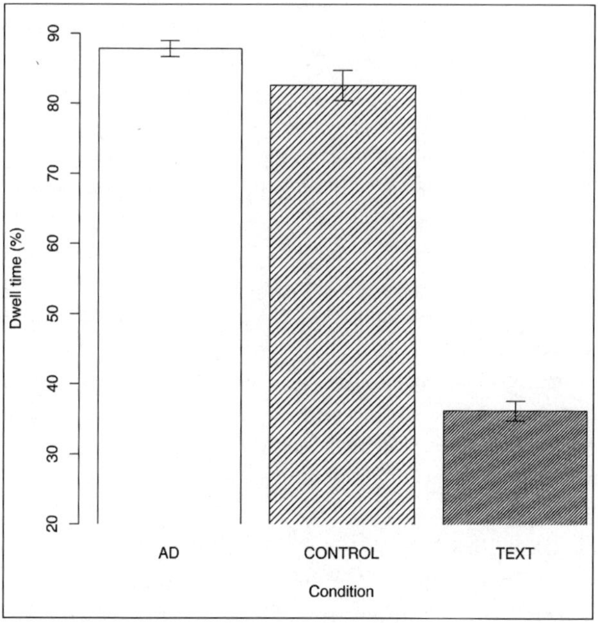

Fig. 12: *Group differences in dwell time on the Caravaggio painting*

These preliminary results are in line with our initial predictions: the AD group focused significantly longer on the painting. What is more, their eye movements followed the description of the painting read by the voice talent. This viewing pattern was markedly different from the other two conditions, which demonstrates that AD guides the viewer's attention towards the elements described in the painting.

We believe that AD can be an attractive aid to developing visual literacy. It can be used in museums, art galleries and educational settings as supplement information broadening young people's art perspectives. Because listening to AD while watching a piece of art employs two different modalities, it leaves some cognitive resources necessary for more thorough visual analysis.

8. Conclusions and future work

In this article we have presented four eye-tracking studies on subtitling for the deaf and hard of hearing and on audio description for the blind and partially sighted as well as sighted people. We hope to have shed some new light on how people watch subtitles and how they perceive audio described works. The results of our research can be implemented in the audiovisual translation professional market practices as well as in education.

Combined with other methods of data collection, such as preference questionnaires or comprehension tests, eye-tracking methodology has proved to be helpful in providing quantitative evidence to testify our hypotheses. However, the application of eye-tracking to audiovisual translation in general and to media accessibility in particular still remains a largely uncharted territory, hampered by the lack of established methodological tools. As rightly noted by J.-L. Kruger (2012: 71), so far most eye-tracking studies on AVT have analysed 'static elements in a dynamic scene and not […] dynamically changing areas of interest'. The application of eye-tracking tools designed for the analysis of static scenes seems inadequate because film is a dynamic medium. In a film, pictures change quickly over time, objects which are being fixated move and so do viewers' eyes. This requires, for instance, an analysis of smooth pursuits, which are not taken into consideration by most eye-tracking studies. The reason for this has naturally stemmed from the technical constraints offered by commercial software available until recently. However, with new software now available on the market it is possible to trace smooth pursuits as part of the dwell time (defined as the total duration of all fixations and saccades in a defined AOI, see J.-L. Kruger 2012) with high-speed eye-trackers.

References

American Council for the Blind (2009): *Audio description standards.* [www.acb.org/dp/docs/DP_Standards.doc].

Caffrey, C. (2012): *Eye-tracking application for measuring the effects of experimental subtitling procedures on viewer perception of subtitled AV content.* In: E. Perego (ed.), Eye-tracking and audiovisual translation. Roma. 225–260 (in press).

Carpenter, P. A./ M. A. Just (1983): *What your eyes do while your mind is reading.* In: K. Rayner (ed.), Eye movements in reading: perceptual and language processes. New York. 275–307.

Chmiel, A./ I. Mazur (2012): *Audio Description Made to Measure: Reflections on Interpretation in AD based on the Pear Tree Project Data.* In: A. Remael/ O. Pilar/ M. Carroll (eds), Audiovisual Translation and Media Accessibility at the Crossroads. Media for All 3. Amsterdam/ New York. 173–188.

Chmiel, A./ I. Mazur/ A. Vilaro/ E. Digiovanni/ P. Chmiel/ P. Orero (2010): *How Audio Description Influences Perception. A Work-In-Progress Report on an International Eye-Tracking Study.* ARSAD 2010.

D'Ydewalle, G./ W. De Bruycker (2007): *Eye Movements of Children and Adults While Reading Television Subtitles.* In: European Psychologist. 12(3). 196–205.

D'Ydewalle, G./ I. Gielen (1992): *Attention allocation with overlapping sound, image, and text*. In: K. Rayner (ed.), Eye movements and visual cognition: Scene perception and reading. New York. 415–427.

D'Ydewalle, G./ J. V. Rensbergen/ J. Pollet (1987): *Reading a message when the same message is available auditorily in another language: The case of subtitling*. In: J. K. O'Reagan/ A. Lévy-Schoen (eds), Eye Movements: From Physiology to Cognition. Amsterdam/ New York. 313–321.

de Linde, Z./ N. Kay (1999): *The semiotics of subtitling*. Manchester.

Duchowski, A. T. (2002): *A breadth-first survey of eye-tracking applications. Behavior Research Methods*. In: Instruments and Computers. 1–16.

d'Ydewalle, G./ C. Praet/ K. Verfaillie/ J. van Rensbergen (1991): *Watching Subtitled Television: Automatic Reading Behaviour*. In: Communication Research. 18(5). 650–666.

Frazier, G./ I. Coutinho-Johnson (1995): *The Effectiveness of Audio Description in Processing Access to Educational AV Media for Blind and Visually Impaired Students in High School*. San Francisco.

Ghia, E. (2012): *The impact of translation strategies on subtitle reading*. In: E. Perego (ed.), Eye-tracking and audiovisual translation. Roma. 155-181.

Hershler, O./ S. Hochstein (2005): *At first sight: A high-level pop-out effect for faces*. In: Vision Research. 45. 1707–1724 (in press).

Irwin, D. E./ G. J. Zelinsky (2002): *Eye Movements And Scene Perception: Memory For Things observed*. In: Perception and Psychophysics. 64. 882–895.

Jensema, C. (1998): *Viewer reaction to different television captioning speeds*. In: American Annals of the Deaf. 143. 318–324.

Jensema, C./ R.S. Danturthi/ R. Burch (2000b): *Time spent viewing captions on television programs*. In: American Annals of the Deaf. 145(5). 464–468.

Jensema, C./ S. E. Sharkawy/ R. S. Danturthi/ R. Burch/ D. Hsu (2000a): *Eye movement patterns of captioned television viewers*. In: American Annals of the Deaf. 145(3). 275–285.

Krejtz, I./ A. Szarkowska/ A. Walczak/ K. Krejtz/ A. Duchowski (2012): *Audio Description as an Aural Guide of Children's Visual Attention: Evidence from an Eye-Tracking Study*. In: ETRA 2012 Proceedings of the Symposium on Eye-tracking Research and Applications, pp. 99-106. ACM New York, NY. [http://dl.acm.org/citation.cfm?doid=2168556.2168572].

Krejtz, K./ I. Krejtz/ A. Duchowski/ A. Szarkowska/ A. Walczak (2012): *Multimodal learning with audio description: an eye-tracking study of children's gaze during a visual recognition task*. In: Proceedings of the ACM Symposium on Applied Perception (SAP '12): ACM, New York, NY, USA, 83-90. DOI=10.1145/2338676.2338694

Kruger, J.-L. (2012): *Making meaning in AVT: eye-tracking and viewer construction of narrative*. In: Perspectives: Studies in Translatology. 20(1), March 2012. 67–86

Langton, S. R. H./ A. S. Law/ A. M. Burton/ S. R. Schweinberger (2008): *Attention capture by faces*. In: Cognition. 107. 330–342.

Majaranta, P./ K.-J. Raiha (2002): *Twenty Years of Eye Typing:Systems and Design Issues*. In: Eye-tracking Research & Applications (ETRA) Symposium. New Orleans, LA.

Mazur, I./ A. Chmiel (2011): *Odzwierciedlenie percepcji osób widzących w opisie dla osób niewidomych. Badania okulograficzne nad audiodeskrypcją*. In: Lingwistyka Stosowana/ Applied Linguistics/ Angewandte Linguistik. 4. 163–180.

Mazur, I./ A. Chmiel (2012): *Towards common European audio description guidelines: results of the Pear Tree Project* In: Perspectives: Studies in Translatology. 20/ 1. 5-23.

Moran, S. (2012): *The effect of linguistic variation on subtitle reception*. In: E. Perego (ed.), Eye-tracking and audiovisual translation. Roma. 183–223 (in press),

Orero, P./ A. Chmiel (forthcoming): *Eye-tracking analysis of minor details in films for audio description*. In: R. Agost/ E. di Giovanni/ P. Orero (eds), Multidisciplinarity in audiovisual translation [Special issue]. MonTi. 4.

Peli, E./ E. M. Fine/ A. T. Labianca (1996): *Evaluating Information Provided By Audio Description*. In: Journal of Visual Impairment and Blindness. 90. 378–385.

Perego, E./ F. de Missier/ M. Porta/ M. Mosconi (2010): *The cognitive effectiveness of subtitle processing*. In: Media Psychology, 13, 243–272.

Rajendran, D. J./ A. T. Duchowski/ P. Orero/ J. Martínez/ P. Romero Fresco (2011): *Effects of text chunking on subtitling: A quantitative and qualitative examination*. [www.andrewd.ces.clemson.edu/research/vislab/docs/perspectives.pdf].

Rayner, K./ S. A. Duffy (1988): *On-line comprehension processes and eye movements in reading*. In: M. Daneman/ G. E. MacKinnon/ T. G. Waller (eds), Reading research: Advances in theory and practice. New York. 13–66.

Rayner, K. (1998): *Eye movements in reading and information processing: Twenty years of research*. In: Psychological Bulletin. 124. 372–422.

Rayner, K./ A. Duffy/ J. Ashby/ Ch. Clifton, Jr (2012): *Psychology of reading, 2nd edition*. New York.

Romero-Fresco, P. (ed) (in press): *The reception of subtitling for the deaf and hard of hearing in Europe*.

Schmeidler, E./ C. Kirchner (2001): *Adding Audio Description: Does It Make a Difference?* In: Journal of Visual Impairment and Blindness. 95(4). 198–212.

Szarkowska, A. (2010): *Accessibility to the Media by Hearing Impaired Audiences in Poland: Problems, Paradoxes, Perspectives*. In: J. Díaz Cintas/ A. Matamala/ J. Neves (eds), New Insights into Audiovisual Translation and Media Accessibility. Media for All 2. Rodopi: Amsterdam/ New York. 139–158.

Szarkowska, A. (2011): *Text-to-speech audio description: towards wider availability of AD*. In: Journal of Specialised Translation. 15. 142–163.

Szarkowska, A./ I. Krejtz/ Z. Kłyszejko/ A. Wieczorek (2011): *Verbatim, standard, or edited? Reading patterns of different captioning styles among deaf, hard of hearing, and hearing viewers*. In: American Annals of the Deaf. 156 (4). 363–378.

Trevarthen, C.B. (1968): *Two mechanisms of vision in primates*. In: Psychologische Forschung. 31. 229–337.

Udo, J.-P./ D. I. Fels (2009): *The Rogue Poster-Children of Universal Design: Closed Captioning and Audio Description*. In: Ted Rogers School of Information Technology Management Publications and Research. Paper 18. http://digitalcommons.ryerson.ca/trsitm/18.

Velichkovsky, B. M./ M. Fels/ J. R. Helmert/ S. Pannasch (2005): *Two Visual Systems and Their Eye Movements: Evidence from Static and Dynamic Scene Perception*. In: CogSci 2005: Proceedings of the XXVII Conference of the Cognitive Science Society. 2283–2288.

Vilaró, A./ P. Orero (forthcoming): *The audio description of leitmotifs*. In: S. Bruti/ E. di Giovanni/ P. Orero (eds), Audio visual translation across Europe: An ever-changing landscape. Bern/ Berlin.

Vilaró, A./ A. Duchowski/ P. Orero/ T. Grindinger/ S. Tetreault/ E. di Giovanni (2012): *How Sound is The Pear Tree Story? Testing the Effect of Varying Audio Stimuli on Visual Attention Distribution*. In: Perspectives: Studies in Translatology 20 (1): Special Issue on The Pear Stories. 55–65.

Walczak, A. (2010): *Audio description for children. A case study of text-to-speech audio description of educational animation series Once Upon a Time... Life* (unpublished MA thesis) [http://avt.ils.uw.edu.pl/files/2012/09/Walczak_TTSAD-for-children.pdf].

Walczak, A./ A. Szarkowska (forthcoming): *Text-to-speech audio description. Testing educational materials with visually-impaired children.*

Yarbus, A. L. (1967): *Eye movements and vision*. New York.

Eye-Tracking Research of Business Email Reception

Justyna Zając (University of Warsaw)

Introduction

The past decade has witnessed a remarkable upsurge of scholarly interest, especially by business communication researchers, in the use of business email. However, there is still far too little knowledge available concerning the effects of email use on business practice, in particular on (in)effective specialist communication, and thus on business success (or failure). Far less is known about business email receipt and, in general, about business email discourse conducted in multinational and global corporations in which work is, to a great extent, undertaken in the form of projects. The study presented in this paper explores selected issues of business email discourse conducted among status equals (project team members) within a global corporation, especially the initiating of business email discourse and the titling of business emails. Therefore, this study contributes to widening our understanding of business email receipt in an intercultural and international business environment.

1. Business email discourse in global project teams: language and culture

Transnational companies usually adopt a geocentric (global) approach to staffing, which means that not only managers but also ordinary employees working for different national offices collaborate on a daily basis. The choice of a geocentric strategy enables top managers to form global virtual teams and thus be competitive and profit in the global market. The selection of this strategy requires the so-called blending/integration of cultures (see E. H. Schein 2009: 13 ff) or, in other words, the formation of a 'professional culture' (see R. Salvi 2011: 22) or a 'third culture' (see K. Knapp 1995: 19, A. Thomas 2003: 44), and the choice of a common language, the so-called 'lingua franca'. More and more companies choose English as the lingua franca for both internal and external communication rather than the national languages used in the particular headquarters (F. Poppi 2011: 235). When adopted in a global business environment, English is usually referred to as 'Business English as a lingua franca' (BELF for short, see L. Louhiala-Salminen/M. Charles/A. Kankaanranta 2005: 403–404). With regard to specific global project teams the concept of 'third culture' and 'third language' may be narrowed to 'team culture' and 'team language' (see J. Zając 2012c), due to the fact that the culture and the language, on which specialist discourse depend, are developed by the given team members for the purposes of the executed project, and they are rarely fully comprehended by members of other project teams. Furthermore, team culture and team language are mostly developed by non-native speakers of English within and for specific contexts, hence non-standard cultural and linguistic forms are developed, which makes it even less easier for other (specialist) speaker-listeners to comprehend these forms and thus participate in the discourse conducted by the given team (see R. Salvi 2011: 30 ff).

1.1. Defining 'project' and 'global virtual teams'

According to the PMBOK Guide (2008: 5), considered an international standard for professionals dealing with project management, 'a project is a temporary endeavor undertaken to create a unique product, service, or result.' Projects need to be distinguished from the company's day-to-day business, as they consist of a one-off set of activities usually undertaken by employees representing different departments of a company. At present, the complexity and interdisciplinary character of projects, together with the expectations of low cost and high quality project outcomes, motivate top managers to form global project teams within one company or in collaboration with external partners. These teams may be called 'global virtual teams' (see N. Zakaria/A. Amelinckx/D. Wilemon 2004). According to N. Zakaria, A. Amelinckx and D. Wilemon (2004: 17),

> [...] global virtual teams are not only separated by time and space, but differ in national, cultural and linguistic attributes, and use information and communication technologies as their primary means of communication and work structure (N. Zakaria/A. Amelinckx/D. Wilemon 2004: 17).

The role of communication in global virtual teams is of the utmost importance (see J. Gimenez 2006: 156–157). In fact, actions taken by members of global virtual teams should mainly be regarded as communicative tasks. Due to the fact that the participants of global virtual teams communicate to a great extent via (business) email (*ibid.* p. 161), in this paper I focus on business email discourse.

1.2. Characteristics of business email discourse

Within the meaning of anthropocentric linguistics (F. Grucza, 1983, 1989, 1992a, 1992b, 1993a, 1993b, 1997, 2010; S. Grucza 2006a, 2006b, 2010, 2011, 2012a, 2012b, 2012c), an email is a text and emails exchanged in professional settings are specialist texts. In this paper, I use the word 'business' instead of 'specialist' due to the fact that the emails analysed for the purposes of this paper were exchanged in a business context. As such, business emails constitute a real means of business communication. Experts produce, send, receive and understand business emails on the basis of their real specialist languages. Realised in a graphic form, business emails represent certain specialist knowledge and specialist information, i.e. business emails are characterised by informative (content) specialty. They are also characterised by expressive specialty, i.e. by terminologicality and certain textual conventions (patterns) used by experts in a given field (here: project management). Both informative and expressive specialty are gradual, as they depend on specialist knowledge produced by specialists and the (cultural) context in which these specialists operate.

Although emails are exchanged in a written form with the help of a computer, smart phone etc., they also resemble the features of spoken language, which J. Gimenez (2000: 239) aptly summarises:

> […] emails combine features of spoken discourse (its nature) with those of written discourse (its representation) to be transmitted or received by a computer.

This observation has also been made by other authors, including F. Poppi (2011: 236), P. Gillaerts (2012: 19–22), N. Van den Eynden Morpeth (2012: 48). The combination of spoken and written discourse features is a result of the unplanned character of emails. At the same time, it implies an informality of business email messages, especially when exchanged between status equals. This may be observed, for instance, through a higher tolerance for mistakes (lexical, orthographical, spelling, punctuation, capitalisation), the use of contracted forms, informal salutations ('Hi' instead of 'Dear'), simple syntactic structures, short sentences, the reliance on the immediate context, and the use of the sender's first name alone (J. Gimenez 2000: 241–248).

Furthermore, (business) emails are characterised by a certain structure. They consist of a header and content (container). On the basis of the header, the information about the sender, subject, date of email receipt, appendices, importance of the email can be reproduced. This type of data appears automatically in the email, when it is forwarded or when one replies to it (see Figure 1).

From: A
Sent: Tuesday, February 01, 2011 6:59 PM
To: X, Y
***CC:** Z
Subject: RE:
***Attachments:** xx.doc, yy.jpg
***Importance:** High

Container

Fig. 1: Email structure (optional elements)*

Added to this, from the automatically constructed structure, the receiver can also find out, if applicable and possible[1], the other addressees of the given email (the lines: 'To:', 'CC:').

On the other hand, the content of an email, the so-called 'container' (J. Bittner 2003: 161), constitutes the real specialist text. It encompasses an unlimited number of characters. The length of specialist texts depends on the specialist-sender. The content is usually composed of the following elements: greeting (salutation), introduction, (proper) container, conclusion, closing, signature (see more Section 3.1.). Moreover, email writers use various formatting options, such as bold, italics, underlining, font colour, font size, lists, in order to make the receiver pay attention to certain words, phrases etc.

Participants of global virtual teams usually exchange (business/specialist) emails, i.e. email writers require email receivers to take certain actions and then to reply to the emails that they have composed and sent to them ('dialogue messages', see A. Kankaanranta 2005: 220; 'To-Do-E-Mails', see S. Voigt 2006: 23–24). Due to the fact that the exchanged business emails are generated in response to one another and thus form a series of connected messages, they are also called 'embedded business emails' (J. Gimenez 2006: 159):

> […] two types of messages make up an embedded email: main messages and subordinate messages which rely on the main messages to make complete sense. The subordinate messages produce a chain which is initiated and finished by the main messages. [...] an embedded email contains a first main message, called the 'chain initiator', which starts the communication process, one or several internal, embedded messages and a final main message, called the 'chain terminator', which brings the event to an end. It should be noted that in embedded emails the chain terminator appears first in the textual chain whereas the chain initiator appears last.

In global virtual teams it is important to keep records of the discourse conducted in order to quickly access 'historical' data concerning mistakes and promises made, deadlines agreed etc. Embedded emails provide the possibility of storing and retrieving data as well as referring to it, if need be, in a highly flexible manner (*ibid.* p. 161). This frequently proves helpful to team members. For these reasons, the supervisors of team members, called project managers, usually forbid them to delete email history.

Taking the above consideration into account, communication via business email may be labelled 'business email discourse' and can be depicted in the following threefold manner (see J. Zając 2012b):

---

1 If the composer has used the blind-copy option ('blind carbon copy', BCC for short), the addressee is not able to see the other email addresses to which the message was sent.

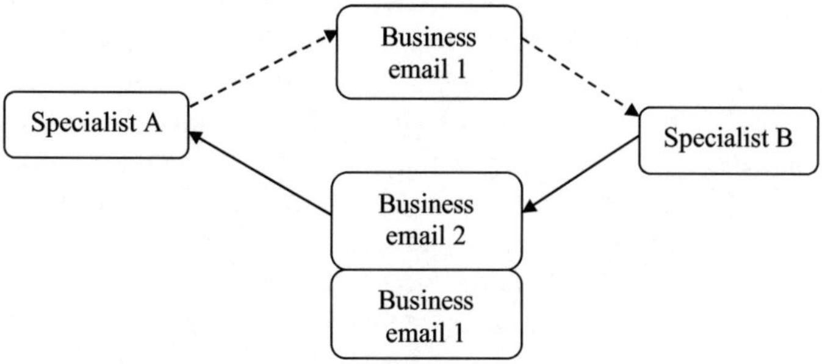

Fig. 2a: Business email discourse

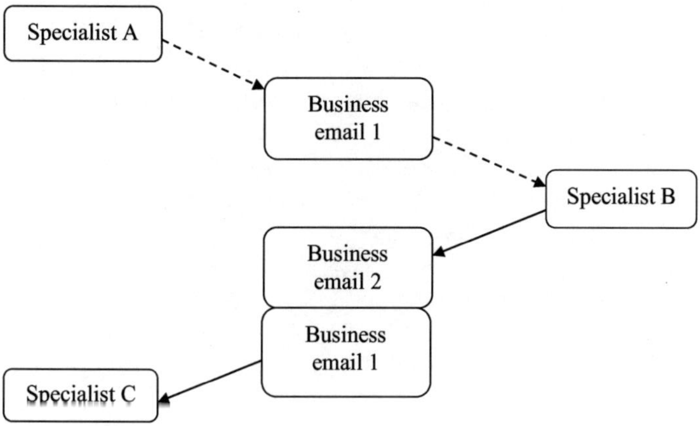

Fig. 2b: Business email discourse

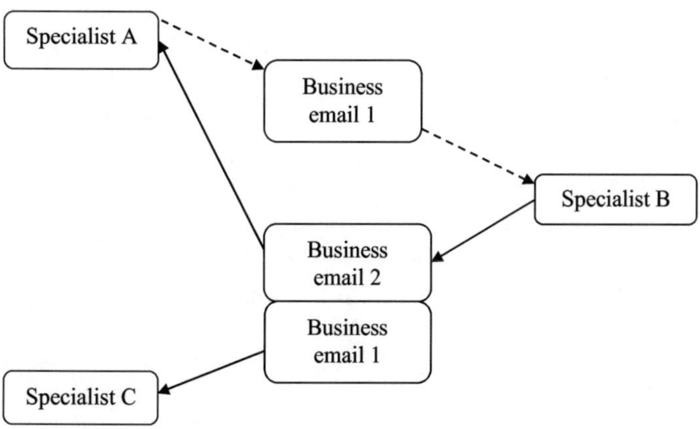

Fig. 2c: Business email discourse

Due to the fact that members of global virtual teams might exchange up to 100 emails daily, it is worth dividing every business email discourse into stages/phases. According to Z. Nęcki (1992: 105 ff) and A. Duszak (1998: 127), we can distinguish three phases of discourse: initial, middle, final. Business emails may play different roles in a given discourse depending on the discourse phase in which they are produced (see A. Deppermann 2008: 58–59). The discourse phases are separated from one another in an explicit or implicit way with the help of the so-called 'boundary markers', which I do not discuss in detail in this paper. The number of phases, as well as the moments at which they begin and end, are usually related to the task at hand (*ibid.* p. 76). The initial (opening) phase and the final (closing) phase of the business email discourse are labelled 'strategic positions' (see A. Duszak 1998: 128) of the business email discourse, constituting its frame. On the other hand, in the middle phase of discourse 'additional' sequences are created. Amongst them we distinguish presequences (which constitute an introduction to the middle phase), postsequences (which summarise the middle phase), inserted sequences (which complement the middle phase), and subsequences (which disrupt the middle phase). The orientation of business email discourse is made easier thanks to the so-called 'mnemotechnical macrostructural signals' (A. Duszak 1998: 128 ff). Amongst these signals we distinguish, above all, the title of discourse and the so-called 'textual means standing out graphically or prosodically'.

In this paper, I discuss the receipt of embedded business emails. Due to the limited space available in this paper, I focus on business email titles and business emails initiating the entire global/local discourses (see 'Specialist email 1', Figures 2a, 2b, 2c). I explicate these issues taking a particular business email discourse under scrutiny.

2. The present study

The present study is part of a larger research project that investigated specialist (business) email communication in a global corporation ('GLOBAL' for short) relying on geographically dispersed (distributed) teams called 'project teams' (here 'global virtual teams', see Section 1.1.). Initially, the detailed findings of the study were presented in my PhD thesis written in Polish, which I later modified, corrected, and translated into English (J. Zając 2012d). In this paper, I present the findings concerning the receipt of emails initiating business email discourse (Section 3.1.) and business email titles (Section 3.2.), which I later compared with the empirical results of the analysis made with eye-tracking measurements.

2.1. Data and email donor

GLOBAL shared 41 authentic emails exchanged by a global virtual team ('Team' for short) composed of four employees deriving from three various countries (Poland, Slovakia, India), i.e. speaking different mother tongues and representing different cultural properties whilst collaborating on a given project. The Team communicated in Business English as a lingua franca, and gradually developed a common team language (see Section 1.2.). For reasons of confidentiality, the name of the email donor and all other names, in particular the employees' names, and identifying information were masked. Moreover, certain parts of selected quotations had to remain undisclosed, therefore I replaced them with square brackets with three dots [. . .]. However, I tried to preserve the original formatting of the quoted texts.

According to GLOBAL's website, the company is the leading provider of predominantly translation and localisation services. It has around 4500 employees working from 26 offices located around the world. For the purposes of the research project, I collaborated directly with the representatives of the Warsaw office ('WAW' for short). GLOBAL adopted a geocentric approach to staffing (see Section 1), which means that the company's offices are managed by local managers who follow the global strategy of the company. However, every local office is independent. Ordinary employees based in all offices communicate directly with one another in English, as it is the mother tongue of the employees located in headquarters and the first foreign language of the majority of the rest of the employees. GLOBAL delivers external projects (i.e. projects for external clients) carried out by global virtual teams consisting of members from various national offices. The participants of global virtual teams perform their duties according to the standards laid down in the PMBOK Guide (2008).

2.2. Methods

In this paper, I focus on the selected findings of business email reception, which I verified on the basis of eye-tracking analysis. Hence, the research project carried out for the purposes of this article consisted of two parts, in which the business emails exchanged by the Team were analysed with the use of the following methods: (1) the traditional qualitative method combining selected elements of ethnographic research, corpus-based method, genre analysis, text analysis and (2) eye-tracking analysis. For the second part of my research, I used the eye-tracker SMI RED 500. With the help of this device, I carried out my experiments at the LELO Eye-Tracking Laboratory[2] and analysed the data using

2 Eye-Tracking Experimental Linguistics Laboratory: www.lelo.uw.edu.pl

the resolution of 120Hz. The experiments were carried out with the use of the original data (no parts of the text were deleted or modified) on three volunteers: Volunteer 1: a former GLOBAL's employee; Volunteer 2: a person with an excellent command of English (Proficiency level, CPE[3] exam), but no previous work experience in a global company; Volunteer 3: a person with a good command of English (TOEFL[4]) and no previous work experience in a global company. I analysed the results using the software SMI BeGaze, which is integrated with the eye-tracker. I would like to emphasise that the analysis using traditional methods (1) was made without prior knowledge of the results of the eye-tracking measurements (2).

In both parts of the project, the tenets of anthropocentric linguistics (of specialist text and discourse, see F. Grucza 2010) constituted the basis of analysis. Briefly, according to anthropocentric linguistics, the aim of the researcher is to reproduce real (specialist) languages (idiolects and polylects), i.e. the linguistic properties of specific specialists and not mental constructs. The researcher concentrates especially on specialists' text-production properties and text-analysis properties, as well as their discursive properties, on the basis of which specialists can produce specialist discourses in an oral/written/hybrid form, and hence participate in textual interactions (F. Grucza 2010: 40 ff). The primary research data consists of real (also 'incorrect and imperfect') texts/discourses available for direct empirical observation and should be analysed within specific contexts and situations (*ibid.* p. 47). Moreover, all indicators appearing in discursive (textual) interaction fulfilling any communicative roles, i.e. para- and extralinguistic indicators and cultural indicators (secondary research data) should also be taken into account when undertaking linguistic analysis (*ibid.* p. 52–53). As a result, linguistic analysis may not only lead, as mentioned above, to the reproduction of the specialists' linguistic properties, but also to the assessment of the state of specialist communication conducted by specific specialists, and to the attempted optimalisation of the given specialist discourse.

3. Data analysis and results

The results section consists of two parts. Firstly, I report on the results of the analysis of business emails initiating two discourses: local and global (Section 3.1.). Secondly, I present the findings concerning those business email titles produced during project execution (Section 3.2.). In both cases I discuss the results of the qualitative analysis in comparison with the findings of the eye-tracking analysis.

3 Certificate of Proficiency in English

4 Test of English as a Foreign Language

3.1. Initiating business email discourse

In project management, the initial phase of business email discourse is critical for two reasons. Firstly, it is the moment at which all the details of the project execution are (or should be) outlined, and thus the initial phase influences the other phases of the discourse. Secondly, it is a starting point for project team members to build interpersonal relationships and communicative equilibrium. However, the initiation phase of business email discourse is subject to certain barriers and limitations due to the fact that there is no direct contact between the team members when they exchange emails (similarly to written communication via letter and oral communication on the telephone or through the door etc., see A. J. Liddicoat 2007: 213, 251). Moreover, the receipt of an email is not sufficient to begin the interaction. According to anthropocentric linguistics, the receiver must have first understood the signal (here business email), which can be observed, for instance, on the basis of the reaction of the addressee to the received email. This also applies to the ringing telephone: ringing may be regarded as summons to the interaction, but it does not mark the beginning of the communication process.

In general, the reception process of a business email initiating the entire business discourse may be divided into two stages: (1) technical and (2) linguistic (see Section 1.2.). The technical stage may be further divided into the following phases: (a) summons to interaction (email receipt) and (b) identification of the sender, subject and the date of the email receipt (email header), whereas within the linguistic stage we may distinguish certain obligatory elements, i.e. (c) greeting (a greeting word); (d) addressing the receiver (by using their first names); (e) description of the task at hand, and optional elements, such as (f) sign off (a closing expression) and (g) name of the specialist-sender (signature).

(1) From a technical point of view, (business) emails may be sent and received with the help of a computer with access to the Internet and a specific software which enables email exchange. Hence, the computer may be labelled the medium of business email discourse. The receiver of an email 'identifies' its receipt visually (and aurally), as a notification of email receipt appears on the computer screen (a). If the given specialist uses loudspeakers, they can also hear that a new email has landed in their inbox. Additionally, the name 'Inbox' is in bold, and beside the Inbox the number of new emails is given in brackets. Every unread email is marked with a closed envelope symbol (in the case of read emails, the sign changes into an open envelope), and the name of the email composer, email subject and the date of its receipt are in bold. Therefore, on the basis of the header (the so-called 'mnemotechnical macrostructural signal', see Section 1.2.) the receiver may go on to the next stage of identification concerning a given email, i.e. the receiver finds out who composed and sent the

email, what its subject is, when the email was received, and whether it was marked as important/urgent (b). The receiver opens the given email by clicking on it. Having opened the message, the receiver also finds out, to whom it was sent (on the condition that the sender has put the email addresses of the receivers in 'To:' or 'CC' lines, and not in the 'BCC' line (*ibid.*)). In project teams, emails are usually sent to a group of people, and the email addresses of the recipients are visible. Moreover, having opened the given email, the receiver may read the content (container, specialist text, *ibid.*).

(2) From a linguistic point of view, a business email is a specialist text (Section 1.2.). In the entire business email discourse under study, two business emails may be regarded as those business emails initiating the discourse. The email presented in Example 1 opened the global discourse, whereas the one in Example 2 initiated the local discourse:

> Hi, DTP and ENG,
>
> Please find the **[. . .]** at the location below:
> FTP address

Example 1: Initiating specialist email discourse (1)

> Hi LPM,
>
> I would like to ask you for [. . .] of below assets for ABCD WLML. **INTL.zip** and **IA.zip** files should be [. . .] for the [. . .] as per attached **[. . .]** file.
> Please, see the further details below:
>
> **Hand off FTP location:**
> **FTP address**
> … look for files **IA.zip** and **INTL.zip**
>
> Above mentioned files **INTL.zip** and **IA.zip** contains:
> **for_translation** folder – **there are RTFs that should be used for [. . .]**
> **logs** folder – where analysis.log file is stored
> **reference** folder – these files should be used **as reference only**
> file **!!!_[. . .] .docx** with instructions how to back convert the [. . .] file into prepared **[. . .].xlsx /[. . .].xlsx**
> ([. . .] RTF and [. . .] XLS should be stored in the same folder; please do not rename these two files because the back conversion will not work properly)
>
> **Hand back FTP location:**
> **FTP address**
>
> **NW location:**
> **FTP address**

… on this location you will find all assets (**including complete wordcounts**) If you have any questions, please let me know. Thank you Best regards ENG

Example 2: Initiating specialist email discourse (2) (the underlined parts of the text were originally given in red font colour)

(c) Both emails started with a greeting. J. Sidnell (2010: 197) observes that greetings are used in order to recognise a person (specialist) whom the sender already knows:

> To greet someone essentially presupposes an already existing relationship of some kind and thus the possibility of mutual recognition. Presumably this is why, if you go up to a stranger on the street and say "hello", they are as likely to give you a cold look and walk away as they are to return the greeting.

This principle does not apply to the context of project management. This may be seen especially when analysing the email presented in Example 1. Although the Team members have not met personally, the project manager greets all team members and uses their names[5]. This (informal) greeting would be impossible in oral communication, e.g. 'face-to-face', if the discourse participants had not met before. In general, greeting presupposes the existence of a personal relationship between the participants of the oral discourse, i.e. the discourse participants must have met before (see e.g. A. Wierzbicka 1999: 58). If the speaker-listeners have not met before, and one of them intends to initiate communication with the other one, then the speaker-listener initiating the discourse usually uses a so-called 'pick-up line', for example the following questions: 'Don't I know you from somewhere?', 'Do you have a light?', 'Do you know when the bus is scheduled to arrive?' (J. Sidnell 2010: 197–198). The greeting presented in Example 1 rarely occurs in email communication, if the emailers have not met before. Generally, when a given person decides to email another person whom they do not know, then after greeting this person they explain the reason for emailing them. However, in specialist email communication conducted by professionals of a given company who have not met before, there is no need for explanations. In addition, no previous personal contact is necessary in order to start the discourse by greeting other team members with the word 'Hi' in tandem

5 In the empirical data, the names of the Team members were replaced with the names of their positions/functions in the projects ('data masking').

with the recipient's name/recipients' names. However, it may be assumed that even though the employees have not met before, a relationship exists between them due to the fact that they work for the same company and collaborate on a common project. It should be emphasised that although the professionals do not know one another properly, they greet one another in an informal way when exchanging specialist emails, not necessarily aiming at building personal relationships. Moreover, in the greetings mentioned above, the distance between Team members is lessened, as they use the word 'Hi'. This word is considered more informal than 'Hello' (A. J. Liddicoat, 2007: 219). However, regardless of which of the mentioned words is used in English, the use of both of them presupposes an already existing relationship between discourse participants (J. Sidnell 2010: 197). As I have mentioned above, the Team members have not met personally before, i.e. they communicate with one another for the first time while conducting the common project. Nevertheless, working for the same company on a project is sufficient to consider the interpersonal relationship to have already been established. Furthermore, the use of the word 'Hi' (instead of 'Hello') in (specialist) email communication is one of the unwritten rules adopted by the employees of the company that shared the data, which is further proof of this company's geocentric approach to staffing. The word 'Hi' is shorter than 'Hello', which may also play a role in the choice of word, especially if the sender composes a considerable number of emails everyday and greets the receiver in every email. Therefore, it may be noted that although Team members communicate with one another for professional reasons (formal context), their discourse is commenced in an informal way and leads to an immediate project start.

(d) Furthermore, the specialist emailer initiating the discourse addresses their colleagues by their first names. According to A. J. Liddicoat (2007: 227), using the first name of a recipient when greeting them (communication on the telephone) undoubtedly displays recognition of a recipient by the speaker. In business email discourse, the use of the first name of a colleague confirms the principle of recipient design, i.e. the given discourse is initiated taking into account other participants:

> […] the fundamental principle of recipient design: the expectation that talk is specifically designed for the particular others who are the recipients (J. Sidnell 2010: 207).

The use of first names of the recipient(s) in business email discourse allows the team members to skip the process of getting to know one another and to reduce the distance between the discourse participants (A. Wierzbicka, 1999: 56 ff), and hence to concentrate on project delivery without any delay. In professional project management, the main goal is to carry out a given project on time and in accordance with the specific guidelines given by the client, and not to establish/develop interpersonal relationships with other team members. However, building interpersonal relationships and reaching communicative equilibrium makes it easier to achieve the common goal. The use of the names of other discourse participants makes them aware of the fact the email that they have received is meant especially for them (it was not sent for their attention only), and that the email composer is awaiting a reply.

(e) The task at hand should be described in great detail in a professional context. However, in the initiation of the global business email discourse (Example 1) we can see that the specialist-sender provided their colleagues merely with a link to certain documents in which the specific guidelines and details were presented. On the other hand, the description of the task in the initiating of the local business email discourse (Example 2) was exhaustive. It is worth pointing out that as a result, the closing of the global business email discourse was more problematic and complicated, whereas the closing of the local business email discourse went quickly and smoothly (see J. Zając 2012d), which may be explained on the basis of the quality of each opening. In the business email initiating the local discourse, the intention to maintain the interaction and carry on with common tasks is more evident. First and foremost, it can be noticed in the length of the email. As opposed to the email in Example 1 (initiating the first phase of the project) consisting of 14 words, the email in Example 2 (initiating the second stage of the project) has 163 words. The specialist-sender also formulates a specific request: 'I would like to ask you for', and then gives the details concerning the work, by using the following expressions (own underlining):

. . . should be . . . as per attached . . . file
Please, see the further details below:
. . . should be stored in . . .; please do not rename . . . because . . . will not work properly.

When describing the details of the task, the specialist-sender uses certain typographic possibilities, particularly bold and two font colours (see Example 2). In this way they let the recipient know which aspects are most relevant and cannot be ignored when delivering the project. In fact, the email in Example 2 may be regarded as instructions (see the underlined parts of sentences above), according to which the specialist-recipient should perform the work. The specialist-sender finishes the email by encouraging the specialist-recipient to communicate in case there are issues to be solved: 'If you have any questions, please let me know'. The sentences presented above help the discourse participants maintain the interaction in a better way than was the case in the email quoted in Example 1. The receiver of the email is encouraged and motivated to discuss problems that may appear during project execution. The specialist-sender also indicates that they know exactly what results they expect. Hence, the detailed description allows the sender not only to motivate the recipient(s) of the email, but also to express their wish that the task is performed in the best possible way.

It is worth paying attention to the optional elements of business emails that I have mentioned above. As regards the sign-off expression (f) used in the emails initiating discourse, the members of the global team under study usually used the expression 'Best regards'. They signed the messages with their first name (g), and they never used their formal signatures with name of their position and full contact information.

When I compared the observations concerning business emails initiating the discourse with the findings of the eye-tracking analysis, I noticed that all subjects focused on the left-hand side of the text, as presented in Figures 4 and 5 (dark gray colour indicating the parts of the greatest gaze fixation during reception of the emails):

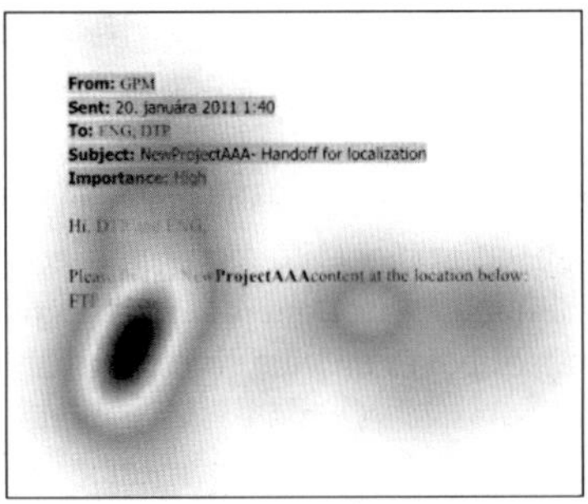

Fig. 4: *Heatmap of the subjects' eye movements as recorded during business email reception (1)*

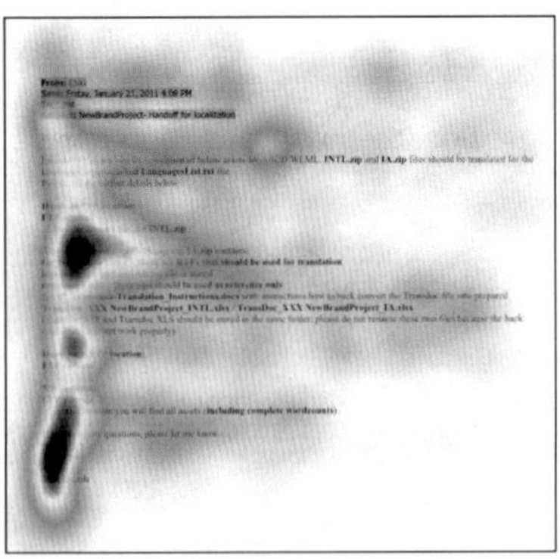

Fig. 5: *Heatmap of the subjects' eye movements as recorded during business email reception (2)*

It is worth explaining that the heatmap depicted in Figure 5 presents the result of the subjects' eye movements registered in two stages. In the first stage, the subjects were asked to imagine working in a global company and being a recipient of the email. They simply read the message. In the second stage, the subjects were asked to answer the email they had just read. In the second stage they could again look at the email while replying to it. During both stages they listened to music, which was playing in the background[6].

Having verified the parts of the business emails the viewers concentrated on as a group, I went on to compare their individual email reception after the first (A) and the second (B) reading of the email (see K. Rayner 1998: 390). The findings were as follows:

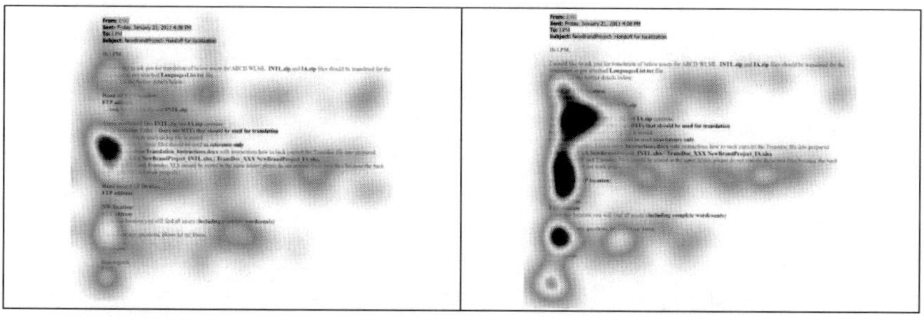

A1 *B1*

Fig. 6: *Heatmap of the eye movements of Volunteer 1 as recorded during business email reception*

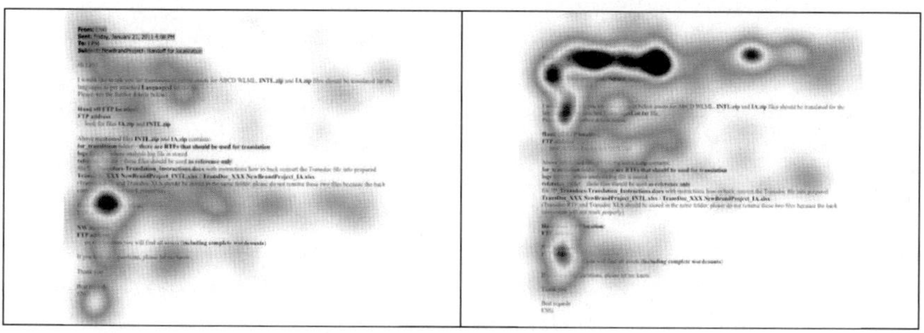

A2 *B2*

6 It is worth mentioning that project team members usually listen to music when working on a given project. Hence, I decided to simulate the real conditions and play music in the background when the experiment was carried out.

Fig. 7: *Heatmap of the eye movements of Volunteer 2 as recorded during business email reception*

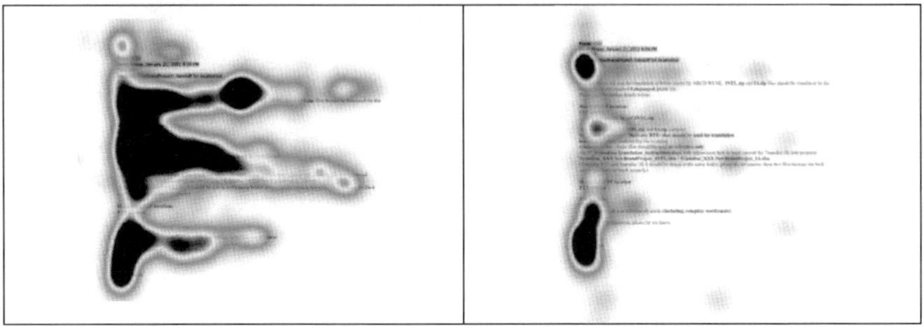

A3 *B3*

Fig. 8: *Heatmap of the eye movements of Volunteer 3 as recorded during business email reception*

It may be observed that during the first reading those volunteers proficient in English scanned the entire email and focused their gaze on the middle part of the email on the left-hand side (A1 and A2). In the second reading, their focus shifted to the middle and final part of the message (B1 and B2). It is worth noting that Volunteer 2, inexperienced in professional settings, paid great attention to the initial part of the email (B2), while the experienced one focused their gaze on the middle and final part of the text (B1). Interestingly, Volunteer 3, whose command of English may be labelled intermediate, read the entire email very carefully during the first reading (A3). Again, greater fixation could be observed on the left-hand-side text. In the second reading, Volunteer 3 scanned the entire email, paying greater attention to the text on the left-hand side (B3). However, the beginning and the end of the message constituted the most interesting points that this person stopped at (the so-called 'entry points'). Therefore, it may be stated that the (fair) effects of font colour and bold were disputed (see K. Rayner 1998: 376). The subjects did not fixate their gaze on the parts of the container exposed with certain typographic options (see also J. Holsanova/H. Rahm/K. Holmqvist 2006: 84–87). They always looked for important information on the left-hand side of the message, which indicates the dark gray colour on the heatmaps in Figures 6, 7 and 8.

3.2. Titles of business emails

During project execution, i.e. when conducting business email discourse, the Team members tended to change the title of the exchanged business emails.

Therefore, I decided to pay closer attention to the email titles as well as to their receipt and influence on the entire business email discourse under study.

In brief, the titles of the emails exchanged by the team members consisted of two parts: the name and number of the project which are usually left unchanged during the entire execution of the project (static part), and the name of the task which must be performed or was performed (dynamic part) which constantly change during the entire project execution. The Team members modified the dynamic part at various stages of the project. However, it is worth pointing out that most of the alterations were introduced in the final phase of the project, both in the static and dynamic part. The modifications in the static part occurred after the project had been listed in a special system and had been given a number, and they were preserved until the end of the project. Conversely, the dynamic part was altered four times in the final phase. All alterations were introduced by one Team member and related to the corrections made to the materials by this Team member. All the changes made in the titles of the business emails were introduced with the help of an underscore, which was followed by appropriate words to indicate the changes:

Modification 1: _X
Modification 2: _Y
Modification 3: _Y_Done
Modification 4: _all [. . .] Updated [. . .]

It should be mentioned that every time a new modification was introduced, the previous one was deleted.

It is worth noting that all modifications to the titles of business emails were short and to the point. On the basis of these the specialist-receiver could easily and quickly, without reading the content, reproduce information on the progress in the project. Therefore, the email titles 'updated' the discourse and were the 'forecaster of global meanings' (see A. Duszak 1998: 129 ff). However, I would like to emphasise that in the discourse under study modifications were not introduced consistently. In addition, the titles of business emails in question were rather chaotic and some words which appeared in them seemed to be redundant, e.g. '[XXX] for [. . .]'. One could use solely the word '[XXX]', as the phrase 'for [. . .]' refers to the activity which was obvious within the context and occurred in all projects conducted in GLOBAL.

At one point, GLOBAL introduced a linguistic rule according to which all emails should be titled in a similar way, as depicted below:

[Project no.] – [Client] – [Project name] – [Department] – TASK

Fig. 9: Model of specialist email titles in project management

Alternatively, specialist emails could be titled in the following way:

Project no. | Client | Project name | Department | TASK

Fig. 9a: *Model of specialist email titles in project management*

By applying one of the above solutions together with the proposed layout (especially by putting the name of the task in capital letters at the end of the title and using square brackets and dashes (Figure 9) or separators (Figure 9a)), the GLOBAL employees could achieve consistency in the titles of specialist emails. Furthermore, adopting one of the models presented in Figures 9 and 9a, would help the members of project teams concentrate on providing only key words in the titles and avoid giving irrelevant information. As a result, the recipient's/recipients' reaction to a given email might be accelerated.

In the eye-tracking experiment, I decided to verify which parts of the email titles human beings focus their attention on. For this reason, I let the subjects see four original titles of the business emails under study, and one theoretical business email title which I formed on the basis of the GLOBAL's guidelines (see Figure 9). As regards the original business email title[7], all viewers concentrated on the first and final part of the email title, which is indicated in the scan path depicted in Figure 10:

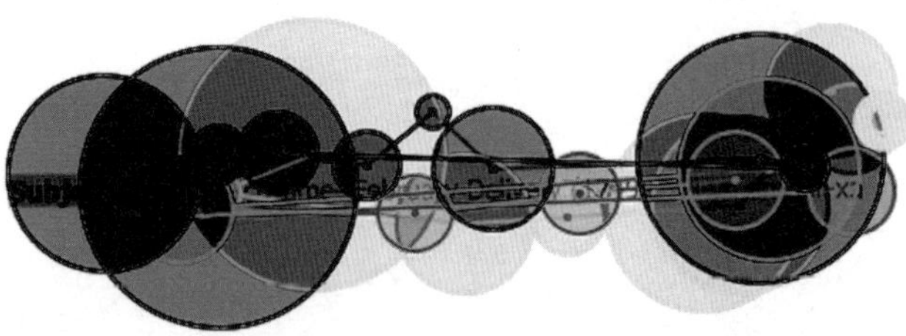

Fig. 10: *Scan path of the subjects' gaze as they viewed the original email title (white smoke colour – Volunteer 1, light gray colour – Volunteer 2, dark gray colour – Volunteer 3)*

On the other hand, in the case of the theoretical business email title[8], the scan path of the gaze looked as such:

7 The selected original business email title looked as follows:
Subject: RE: ProjectName- February Delivery (17498)_vi-vn and ar-xa

8 The theoretical business email title looked as follows:
Subject: [17498] – [Microsoft] – [ProjectName] – [DTP] – CORRECTING FILES

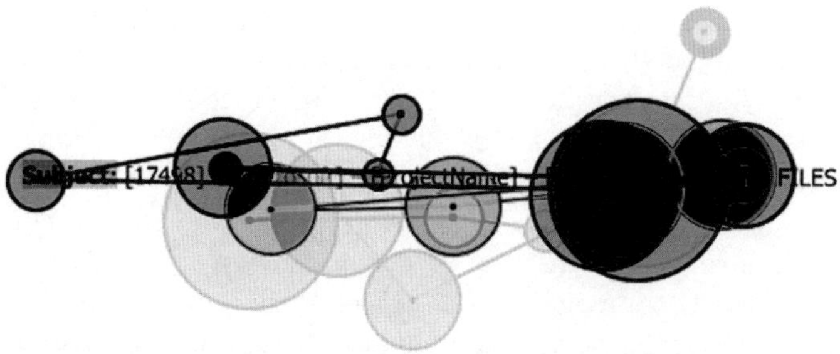

Fig. 11: *Scan path of the subjects' gaze as they viewed the theoretical email title (white smoke colour – Volunteer 1, light gray colour – Volunteer 2, dark gray colour – Volunteer 3)*

On the basis of the Figures 10 and 11, it could be stated that the company's suggestion to put the most relevant words in capital letters at the end of the email title creates the expected results (K. Rayner 1998: 376). In other words, specialist-recipients concentrate mainly on the last words of the email title if they are written in capital letters and the rest of the words are put into order in square brackets. Therefore, adopting the GLOBAL's proposal may indeed speed up the process of email receipt and subsequent reaction (response) to the given email.

4. Discussion

Taking into consideration the results of the eye-tracking analysis presented in Section 3.1., the findings of the study conducted by J. Holsanova, H. Rahm and K. Holmqvist (2006) can be confirmed. The authors made certain assumptions about newspaper reading and verified these using eye-tracking data from readers' actual interaction with a newspaper. According to their results, we can distinguish three main categories of reading behaviour (see also Rayner 1998: 392 ff) and differentiate between editorial readers, overview readers and focused readers. Even though the authors' results apply mostly to (national) newspaper reading and cannot fully be adopted to (business) emails exchanged in international settings, certain reading-behaviour patterns could be noticed in the study presented in this paper. In the first reading, Volunteer 3 devoted their attention to the entire article, as can be observed both on the heatmap result (A3) and by the time frame (1:48.579≈1 minute 50 seconds spent on reading as compared with 40.049 (A1) and 31.709 (A2)), and is therefore labelled 'the focused reader'. In the second reading, Volunteer 3 focused on the most important entry points (the beginning and end of the message) and hence may be called an 'entry-point overviewer'. This can also be confirmed on the basis of the time span devoted to looking at the email: 45.481 (B3) as compared with 1:20.727 (B1) and 2:15.75 (B2). The other two subjects can be labelled 'scanning readers'[9] in the first reading, as they seemed to be going through the email and surmising what it was all about. However, having been told to imagine that they are the recipient of the email, in the second reading they rested their eyes on particular parts (entry points) of the text in order to intake information. Thus, in the second reading they may be labelled 'entry-point overviewers'.

Another interesting issue concerns the layout of a business email and its title. Professional emailers are usually encouraged (according to the GLOBAL's guidelines) to highlight important parts of their texts, using different font colour and size, bold, italics, making lists etc. However, it turns out that email recipients do not necessarily fixate their gaze on these exposed fragments. Interestingly, they concentrate on the left-hand side of emails, and so the effects of layout are disputed. Therefore, it may be beneficial to improved email reception if specialist-senders highlight the most important words and sentences by putting them on the left-hand side of the container. Conversely, email composers should pay attention to the layout of their titles. As it could be seen from the eye-tracking analysis (see Section 3.2.), email-recipients fixate their gaze particularly on the last words of the title, most probably due to the fact that these words are given in capital letters.

5. Conclusions

Before formulating the concluding remarks, I would like to stress that this study, the results of which are presented in this paper, is a small-scale study. It has been limited to a specific method of managing organisations (global project management), to a particular line of business and to a single company. Therefore, the findings should be considered tentative rather than universal and constitute a basis for future research. Nevertheless, certain general statements can be formulated.

9 I prefer to use the term 'scanning reader' instead of 'editorial reader' proposed by J. Holsanova, H. Rahm and K. Holmqvist (2006), as the latter refers more to journalism than to a business context.

Having advocated an anthropocentric approach to linguistic research for some time now, I would like to highlight that the evidence provided by the present study testifies to applying the anthropocentric theory to specialist (business) communication research (see also another study concerning politeness in specialist email discourse in J. Zając 2012a; other studies in which this theory has been successfully applied: S. Bonacchi 2011, 2012; M. Płużyczka 2011a, 2011b, 2012a, 2012b, 2012c). The analysis has revealed that human beings (specialists) receive emails in different ways. In fact, we can distinguish various reading behaviours, such as focused-readers, scanning readers, entry-point overviewers, at different stages of business email reception. Different patterns of business email receipt, which were analysed on the basis of the email initiating a given business email discourse, were related to the subjects' various professional experience and different command of English.

In general, (business) email readers fixate their gaze on the left-hand side of the text. Therefore, sentences and words presenting new/important ideas should be introduced in a new line on the left-hand side of texts. The layout does not seem to play any particular role, as opposed to business email titles. The titles of the emails should be put into order in such a way as the most relevant piece of information is given at the end of the title (right-hand side), preferably in capital letters.

Ultimately, I would like to reiterate that further studies on business email reception should be conducted to make representatives of (transnational) companies and their employees aware of the influence of the practices that they apply. For instance, it would be interesting to verify on which parts of the emails discourse participants concentrate in the middle phase of business discourse. In addition, with the help of eye-tracking measurements it would be important to check if and how politeness expressions influence business discourse. Analysis should also be carried out with regard to specialists representing various linguistic and cultural properties, as doing business internationally is common practice nowadays. Only in this way can reliable tips and training programmes for employees be prepared so that they can develop their email-receptive skills and be better equipped to take advantage of these skills in a business environment.

Acknowledgements

1. The author would like to thank Professor Sambor Grucza for his initial encouragement with this paper.
2. The first part of the study described in this chapter was substantially co-funded by the Systemic Project grant entitled Scientific Potential for the Economy of

Mazovia – Scholarships for PhD Students, co-financed by the European Social Fund and the national public resources contribution under the Sub-measure 8.2.2 of the Human Capital Operational Programme 2007–2013.

HUMAN CAPITAL
NATIONAL COHESION STRATEGY

EUROPEAN UNION
EUROPEAN
SOCIAL FUND

References

Bittner, J. (2003): *Digitalität, Sprache, Kommunikation. Eine Untersuchung zur Medialität von digitalen Kommunikationsformen und Textsorten und deren varietätenlinguistischer Modellierung*. Berlin.

Bonacchi, S. (2011): *Höflichkeitsausdrücke und anthropozentrische Linguistik*. Warszawa.

Bonacchi, S. (2012): *Anthropozentrische Kulturologie: einige Überlegungen zu Grundannahmen und Forschungspraxis anhand der Analyse von Komplimenten*, In: F. Grucza/ P. Zimniak/ G. Pawłowski (eds), Die deutsche Sprache, Kultur und Literatur in polnisch-deutscher Interaktion. Beiträge der internationalen wissenschaftlichen Konferenz des Verbandes Polnischer Germanisten, 17.–19. Juni 2011, Zielona Góra. Warszawa. 33–52.

Deppermann, A. (2008): *Gespräche analysieren*, 4th ed. Wiesbaden.

Duszak, A. (1998): *Tekst, dyskurs, komunikacja międzykulturowa*. Warszawa.

Gillaerts, P. (2012): *E-mail Use un a Belgian Company: Looking for the Hybridity of the Genre*, In: P. Gillaerts/ E. de Groot/ S. Dieltjens/ P. Heynderickx/ G. Jacobs (eds), Researching Discourse in Business Genres. Cases and Corpora. Frankfurt/ M. etc. 15–31.

Gimenez, J. (2000): *Business e-mail communication: some emerging tendencies in register*. In: English for Specific Purposes. 19. 237–251.

Gimenez, J. (2006): *Embedded business emails: Meeting new demands in international business communication*. In: English for Specific Purposes. 25. 154–172.

Grucza, F. (1983): *Zagadnienia metalingwistyki. Lingwistyka – jej przedmiot, lingwistyka stosowana*. Warszawa.

Grucza, F. (1989): *Język a kultura, bilingwizm a bikulturyzm: lingwistyczne i glottodydaktyczne aspekty interlingwalnych i interkulturowych różnic oraz zbieżności*. In: F. Grucza (ed.), Bilingwizm, bikulturyzm, implikacje glottodydaktyczne. Warszawa. 9–49.

Grucza, F. (1992a): *Kulturowe determinanty języka oraz komunikacji językowej*. In: F. Grucza (ed.), Język, kultura – kompetencja kulturowa. Warszawa. 9–70.

Grucza, F. (1992b): *O komunikacji międzyludzkiej – jej podstawach, środkach, rodzajach, płaszczyznach, składnikach i zewnętrznych uwarunkowaniach*. In: W. Woźniakowski (ed.), Modele komunikacji międzyludzkiej. Warszawa. 9–30.

Grucza, F. (1993a): *Język, ludzkie właściwości językowe, językowa zdolność ludzi*. In: J. Piontek/ A. Wierczyńska (eds), Człowiek w perspektywie ujęć biokulturowych. Poznań. 151–171.

Grucza, F. (1993b): *Zagadnienia ontologii lingwistycznej: O językach ludzkich i ich (rzeczywistym) istnieniu.* In: Opuscula Logopaedica. In honorem Leonis Kaczmarek. Lublin. 25–47.

Grucza, F. (1997): *Języki ludzkie a wyrażenia językowe, wiedza a informacja, mózg a umysł ludzki.* In: F. Grucza/ M. Dakowska (eds), Podejście kognitywne w lingwistyce, translatoryce i glottodydaktyce. Warszawa. 7–21.

Grucza, F. (2010): *Od lingwistyki wyrazu do lingwistyki tekstu i dyskursu: o wielości dróg rozwoju lingwistyki i kryteriów jego oceny.* In: A. Waszczuk-Zin (ed.), Publikacja jubileuszowa III. Lingwistyka stosowana – języki specjalistyczne – dyskurs zawodowy. Warszawa. 13–56.

Grucza, S. (2006a): *Idiolekt specjalistyczny – idiokultura specjalistyczna – interkulturowość specjalistyczna.* In: J. Lewandowski/ M. Kornacka/ W. Woźniakowki (eds), Języki specjalistyczne 6. Teksty specjalistyczne w kontekstach międzykulturowych i tłumaczeniach. Warszawa. 30–49.

Grucza, S. (2006b): *Komunikacja specjalistyczna a idiokontekst specjalistyczny i konsytuacja specjalistyczna.* In: Studia Rossica XVIII. Glottodydaktyka i jej konteksty interkulturowe. Warszawa. 209–223.

Grucza, S. (2010): *Główne tezy antropocentrycznej teorii języków.* In: Lingwistyka Stosowana/ Applied Linguistics/ Angewandte Linguistik. 2. 41–68.

Grucza, S. (2011): *Lingwistyka antropocentryczna a badania okulograficzne.* In: Lingwistyka Stosowana / Applied Linguistics / Angewandte Linguistik. 4. 149–162.

Grucza, S. (2012a): *Fachsprachenlinguistik.* Frankfurt/ M.

Grucza, S. (2012b): *Grundzüge der Anthropozentrischen Translatorik.* In: Linguistica Silesiana. An international journal of linguistic studies. (in press).

Grucza, S. (2012c): *Heat maps, gaze plots . . . and what next? The access to translation competences and translation processes* In: S. Grucza/ M. Płużyczka/ J. Zając (eds), Translation Studies and Eye Tracking Analysis. Frankfurt/ M. (in press).

Holsanova, J./ H. Rahm/ K. Holmqvist (2006): *Entry points and reading paths on newspaper spreads: comparing a semiotic analysis with eye-tracking measurements.* In: Visual Communication. 5(1). 65–93.

Kankaanranta, A. (2005): *English as a corporate language: Company-internal email messages written by Finns and Swedes.* In: B. L. Gunnarsson (ed.), Communication in the Workplace, Uppsala, Universitetstryckeriet. 42–59.

Knapp, K. (1995): *Interkulturelle Kommunikationsfähigkeit als Qualifikationsmerkmal für die Wirtschaft.* In: J. Bolten (ed.), Cross Culture – Interkulturelles Handeln in der Wirtschaft. Sternenfels. Berlin. 8–23.

Liddicoat, A. J. (2007): *An Introduction to Conversation Analysis.* London/ New York.

Louhiala-Salminen, L./ M. Charles/ A. Kankaanranta (2005): *English as a lingua franca in Nordic corporate mergers: Two case companies.* In: English for Specific Purposes. 24. 401–421.

Nęcki, Z. (1992): *Komunikowanie interpersonalne.* Wrocław, Warszawa, Kraków.

Płużyczka, M. (2011a): *Eye-Tracking Analysen in der Translationswissenschaft. Zum Stand der Forschung.* In: Kwartalnik Neofilologiczny. LVIII. 4/ 2011. 473–484.

Płużyczka, M. (2011b): *Okulograficzne wsparcie badań nad procesem tłumaczenia a vista.* In: Lingwistyka Stosowana/ Applied Linguistics/ Angewandte Linguistik. 4. 180–189.

Płużyczka, M. (2012a): *Na co patrzy, a co widzi tłumacz a vista? Okulograficzne pytania translatoryki.* In: Lingwistyka Stosowana/ Applied Linguistics/ Angewandte Linguistik. 5. 65–74.

Płużyczka, M. (2012b): *Eye-tracking Support of Translation Processes Analysis*. In: Vestnik MGLU (in press).

Płużyczka, M. (2012c): *Eye-tracking supported research into sight translation. Lapsological conclusions*. In: S. Grucza/ M. Płużyczka/ J. Zając (eds), Translation Studies and Eye-Tracking Analysis. Frankfurt/ M. (in press).

PMBOK Guide (2008): *A Guide to the Project Management Body of Knowledge (PMBOK® Guide)*, 4th ed. Pennsylvania, Project Management Institute, Inc.

Poppi, F. (2011): *Mediating between Local and Global Practices: the Use of English as the Lingua Franca for Internal Company Communications,* In: R. Salvi/ H. Tanak (eds), *Intercultural Interactions in Business and Management*. Bern etc. 235–255.

Rayner, K. (1998): *Eye Movements in Reading and Information Processing: 20 Years of Research.* In: Psychological Bulletin. Vol. 124. No. 3. 372–422.

Salvi, R. (2011): *Changes, Chances and Challanges in Describing Intercultural Professional Interactions,* In: R. Salvi/ H. Tanak (eds), *Intercultural Interactions in Business and Management*. Bern etc. 21–44.

Schein, E. H. (2009): *The Corporate Culture Survival Guide*. San Francisco/ Jossey-Bass.

Sidnell, J. (2010): *Conversation Analysis. An Introduction*. Singapore.

Thomas, A. (2003): *Das Eigene, das Fremde, das Interkulturelle*. In: A. Thomas/ E.-U. Kinast/ S. Schroll-Machl (eds), Handbuch Interkulturelle Kommunikation und Kooperation. Band 1: Grundlagen und Praxisfelder. Göttingen. 44–59.

van den Eynden Morpeth, N. (2012): *Politeness and Gender in Belgian Organisational Emails*. In: P. Gillaerts/ E. de Groot/ S. Dieltjens/ P. Heynderickx/ G. Jacobs (eds), Researching Discourse in Business Genres. Cases and Corpora. Frankfurt/ M. etc. 33–51.

Voigt, S. (2003): *E-Mail-Kommunikation in Organisationen. Eine explorative Studie zu individuellen Nutzungsstrategien*. München.

Wierzbicka, A. (1999): *Język –umysł – kultura. Wybór prac pod redakcją Jerzego Bartmińskiego*. Warszawa.

Zając, J. (2012a): *Specialist Email Communication in Global Virtual Teams: Selected Facets of Politeness*. (11th Annual Conference of the European Association of Languages for Specific Purposes: "The Role of Applied Languages in Tertiary Education in the post – Bologna scenario: boosting autonomy and mobility in a globalised world?" (in press).

Zając, J. (2012b): *Linguistic Issues of Email Discourse in Business Communication*. In: Studia Germanica Gedanensia. 26. 235–246.

Zając, J. (2012c): *Towards Successful Communication in Global Virtual Teams: Team Language and Team Culture*. In: Kwartalnik Neofilologiczny. LIX. 3/ 2012. 345–370.

Zając, J. (2012d): *Communication in Global Corporations. Successful Project Management via Email*. Frankfurt/ M. (forthcoming).

Zakaria, N./ A. Amelinckx/ D. Wilemon (2004): *Working Together Apart? Building a Knowledge-Sharing Culture for Global Virtual Teams*. In: Creativity and Innovation Management. 13/ 1. 15–29.

Notes on Contributors

Prof. Dr. habil. **Sambor Grucza** is Professor at the University of Warsaw, Director of the Institute of Anthropocentric Linguistics and Culturology, Head of the Linguistics of Languages for Specific Purposes Department, Founder and Research Head of the Eye-Tracking Experimental Linguistics Laboratory. He is also Editorial Head of the *Lingwistyka Stosowana/Applied Linguistics/Angewandte Linguistik*, *Studi@ Naukowe* and *Warschauer Studien zur Germanistik und Angewandten Linguistik*. He is President of the *Polish Association of Applied Linguistics*, and the executive board member of the *Polnischer Germanisten Verband* and also a member of several other international academic associations. His research interests are: metalinguistics, text and discourse linguistics, translation studies, translation teaching, glottodidactics, and linguistics of languages for specific purposes. He is currently the head of three international research projects. He is the author of over 120 publications and co-author of 35 text books in the series *Dein Deutsch* for the study of German as a second language. E-mail: sfgrucza@uw.edu.pl, website: www.lelo.uw.edu.pl.

Prof. Dr. **Silvia Hansen-Schirra** is Professor for English linguistics and translation studies at the translation department of the Mainz University in Germersheim (Germany). Her main research interests include empirical translation studies, machine translation and specialized communication. During her PhD, she worked at the computational linguistics department and the translation department of the Saarland University in Saarbrücken (Germany). Her PhD thesis was concerned with the product- and process-oriented investigation of the specific nature of translations. She was the principal investigator of several projects in the field of empirical linguistics and translation studies. Currently she is involved in the investigation of specialized communication and translation on the basis of multi-layer corpus analyses and cognitive experiments. She is the co-editor of the online journal "Translation: Computation, Corpora, Cognition".

Andrew Duchowski, PhD, is Professor of Computer Science at Clemson University. He received his baccalaureate (1990) from Simon Fraser University, Burnaby, Canada, and doctorate (1997) from Texas A&M University, College Station, TX, both in Computer Science. His research and teaching interests include visual attention and perception, eye-tracking, computer vision, and computer graphics. He joined the School of Computing faculty at Clemson in January, 1998. He has since produced a corpus of publications and a textbook related to eye-tracking research, and has delivered courses and seminars on the subject at international conferences. He maintains Clemson's eye-tracking laboratory and teaches a regular course on eye-tracking methodology attracting students from a variety of disciplines across campus.

Izabela Krejtz received her PhD in social psychology from the Institute of Psychology, Polish Academy of Sciences. She is Assistant Professor at the University of Social Sciences and Humanities in Warsaw, Poland. Her research interests include neurocognitive and educational psychology. Her applied work focuses on controlled attention trainings, eye-movements studies in perception of audio visual material and emotions regulation. E-mail: ikrejtz@swps.edu.pl, website: iza.krejtz.org.

Krzysztof Krejtz, PhD, is Assistant Professor at the Department of Psychology, University of Social Sciences and Humanities, and Head of the Interactive Technologies Laboratory at the Information Processing Institute, Warsaw (LABi, www.labi.opi.org.pl). His research interests include visual attention, eye-tracking, Human-Computer Interaction, psychological and social aspects of the Internet, social psychology, statistics and social and cognitive science methodology. He is the author of many publications concerning social aspects of human social life on internet and in context of new media, e.g. *Diagnosis of Internet*, *Internet Culture of Insult*. He is a member of Association of Computing Machinery (ACM) and Social Psychology Association (SPS).

Marta Małachowicz, PhD, is Assistant Professor at the Institute of Anthropocentric Linguistics and Culturology at the University of Warsaw. She graduated from the Faculty of Applied Linguistics, Warsaw University. Her research interests include discourse analysis, terminology and corpus linguistics. Her recent research project included examining methods of terminology management on the example of terminology centers in the Nordic countries (Sweden, Finland). Currently she is working on a project of applying the results of terminology work in teaching languages for specific purposes (LSP) and specialist text translation. She is Assistant to the President of Polish Association of Applied Linguistics. She delivers courses in translation and Russian language. She also works as a freelance translator. E-mail: m.malachowicz@uw.edu.pl.

Monika Płużyczka, PhD, is Assistant Professor at the Institute of Anthropocentric Linguistics and Culturology at the University of Warsaw. She received her doctorate (2009) from the University of Warsaw for her PhD thesis on psycholinguistic aspects of translation teaching. She is Head of the Eye-Tracking Experimental Linguistics Laboratory, Deputy Director of International Affairs at the Institute of Anthropocentric Linguistics and Culturology, Deputy

Editor of *Lingwistyka Stosowana/Applied Linguistics/Angewandte Linguistik* and *Kwartalnik Neofilologiczny* and a member of several international scientific associations. Her research interests include translation studies, especially eye-tracking analyses of translational processes, translation and interpreting teaching. She is currently involved in 3 international research projects on translation. She has also been visiting Assistant Professor at Universities in Moscow, Verona and Pavia. She was awarded several post-doctoral research scholarships in Poland and Germany. E-mail: mpluzyczka@uw.edu.pl, website: www.lelo.uw.edu.pl.

Prof. Dr. **Christoph Rösener** is Professor for international technical communication at the Department of Information and Communication at the Flensburg University of Applied Sciences (Germany). His main research interests include terminology science, language engineering, specialized translation and translation technology. During his PhD, he worked at the Institute of the Society for the Promotion of Applied Information Sciences (IAI) and the Translation Department of Saarland University, both Saarbrücken (Germany). His PhD thesis was concerned with natural language interfaces as a possibility to access knowledge data bases. He was involved in several research projects in the field of machine translation, automatic indexation and classification, mono- and multilingual information retrieval and controlled language authoring tools. Currently he is the principal investigator of a language technology project concerning the use of controlled language checkers in e-learning applications. He is a member of several academic associations and professional bodies.

Paweł Soluch, Neuropsychologist, research worker at the Medical University of Warsaw, scholar of the Foundation for Polish Science, Research Head of the Institute of Sensory Analysis, President of the Board at the *Neuro Device Group* company which specializes in implementing state-of-the-art technologies in behavioral laboratories, lecturer of I Faculty of Medicine at the Medical University of Warsaw, Faculty of Health Sciences at the Medical University of Warsaw and Faculty of Psychology at the University of Warsaw. He was employed for seven years at the Department of Neurosurgery of the Medical University of Warsaw where he specialized particularly in functional neuroimaging (fMRI, DTI, etc.). He is the author and leader of many research projects in neuroimaging, psychophysiology and medicine. Since 2008 he has been operating within the area of eye-tracking. His research interests are: neuroimaging, particularly in relation to smell and taste, as well as eye-tracking and psychophysiology.

Agnieszka Szarkowska, PhD, is Assistant Professor at the Institute of Applied Linguistics at the University of Warsaw. She is the founder and head of the Audiovisual Translation Lab (AVT Lab, www.avt.ils.uw.edu.pl). Her research interests include audiovisual translation, especially subtitling for the deaf and hard of hearing and audio description. Her recent research projects include an eye-tracking study on subtitling for the deaf and hard of hearing, multilingualism in subtitling, audio description in education, text-to-speech audio description, and audio description to foreign films. She is a member of European Association for Studies in Screen Translation and an honorary member of the Polish Audiovisual Translators Association (STAW). She also works as a freelance subtitler and certified translator. Website: www.ils.uw.edu.pl/388.html.

Prof. Dr. habil. **Adam Tarnowski**, is Professor at the University of Warsaw. He graduated in psychology from Akademia Teologii Katolickiej (now Cardinal Stefan Wyszyński University in Warsaw) in 1989. He earned his PhD at the Jagiellonian University (1998) and habilitation at the University of Warsaw (2010) based on the monograph "Working memory and mechanisms of eye movements: 300 milliseconds of human life". His research activity is focused on the relationship between perception and higher level of information processing. At the University of Warsaw he teaches research methodology, statistics, work psychology and ergonomics. He is also the head of postgraduate studies in Transport Psychology. In addition, he is the head of the Department of Aviation Psychology in Military Institute of Aviation Medicine. He is the author or co-author of 70 scientific publications.

Justyna Zając, PhD, is Assistant Professor at the Institute of Culturology and Anthropocentric Linguistics at the University of Warsaw. She received her doctorate (2012) from the University of Warsaw for her PhD thesis on 'Specialist Communication in Global Corporations'. Her main research interests lie in intercultural business and specialist communication, communication in virtual project teams, the use of English as the business lingua franca (BELF) and communications audit. Specialist email discourse is an important topic of her publications. She is a member of the Eye-Tracking Experimental Linguistics Laboratory (www.lelo.uw.edu.pl), Deputy Editor of *Lingwistyka Stosowana/Applied Linguistics/Angewandte Linguistik* and *Kwartalnik Neofilologiczny*. She is also a member of the *Polish Association of Applied Linguistics*, *Internationale Vereinigung für Germanistik, Polnischer Germanisten Verband.* She has been awarded several research scholarships, both national and international. E-mail: justyna.zajac@uw.edu.pl, website: www.lelo.uw.edu.pl.

Ewa Zwierzchoń-Grabowska, PhD, is Assistant Professor at the Institute of Anthropocentric Linguistics and Culturology at the University of Warsaw. She received her doctorate (2006) from the University of Warsaw for her PhD thesis on "Internet. Theoretical model of Internet-based glottodidactic process" and she continues her interests in Internet-based foreign language learning and teaching. Now, her main research interests lie in computer-assisted translation and applications of video eye-tracking in translation studies. She is a member of the Eye-Tracking Experimental Linguistics Laboratory. She is also a member of the *Polish Association of Applied Linguistics* and *Verband Polnischer Germanisten*. E-mail: e.zwierzchon@uw.edu.pl, website: www.lelo.uw.edu.pl.

Prof. Dr. habil. **Jerzy Żmudzki**, is Professor at University of Maria Curie-Skłodowska in Lublin, Founder and Head of the Department of Applied Linguistics and Research Head of Interpreting Studies and Interpreting Teaching Labolatory. He is Vice President of the *Polnischer Germanisten Verband* and the *Polish Association of Applied Linguistics*. He is also a member of the editorial board of *Lingwistyka Stosowana/Applied Linguistics/Angewandte Linguistik* and *Lubelskie Materiały Neofilologiczne*. His research interests are: pragmatics, text linguistic, textlological genenology and translation studies (theory of translation, sight translation, conference and simultaneous interpreting, translation teaching. He is currently involved in some research projects on translation according to (a) experimental based modeling of sight translation, (b) evaluation of multimodal auto description by sight translation, (c) teaching of conference interpreting and sight translation. Website: www.umcs.lublin.pl/lingwistyka_stosowana.

Warschauer Studien zur Germanistik und zur Angewandten Linguistik

Herausgegebenvon Sambor Grucza und Lech Kolago

Band 1 Sambor Grucza: Fachsprachenlinguistik. 2012.

Band 2 Paweł Bąk: Euphemismen des Wirtschaftsdeutschen aus Sicht der anthropozentrischen Linguistik. 2012.

Band 3 Der Mensch und seine Sprachen. Festschrift für Professor Franciszek Grucza. Herausgegeben von Magdalena Olpińska-Szkiełko, Sambor Grucza, Zofia Berdychowska und Jerzy Żmudzki. Unter Mitarbeit von Ewa Bartoszewicz, Monika Płużyczka und Justyna Zając. 2012.

Band 4 Urszula Topczewska: Konnotationen oder konventionelle Implikaturen? 2012.

Band 5 Agnieszka Szarkowska: Forms of Address in Polish-English Subtitling. 2013.

Band 6 Sambor Grucza / Monika Płużyczka / Justyna Zając (eds): Translation Studies and Eye-Tracking Analysis. 2013.

www.peterlang.de